WORKBOOK TO ACCOMPANY

AN INTEGRATED APPROACH TO HEALTH SCIENCES

Anatomy and Physiology, Math, Chemistry, and Medical Microbiology

Second Edition

Bruce J. Colbert, M.S., R.R.T.
and
Jeff Ankney, B.S., R.R.T.
Joe Wilson, B.S., M.S.
John Havrilla, B.S., M.Ed., M.A.

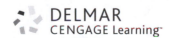

DELMAR
CENGAGE Learning™

Australia • Brazil • Japan • Korea • Mexico • Singapore • Spain • United Kingdom • United States

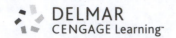
DELMAR
CENGAGE Learning™

Workbook to Accompany *An Integrated Approach to Health Sciences: Anatomy and Physiology, Math, Chemistry, and Medical Microbiology*, **Second Edition**
Bruce J. Colbert, Jeff Ankney, Joe Wilson, John Havrilla

Vice President, Career and Professional Editorial: Dave Garza

Director of Learning Solutions: Matthew Kane

Acquisitions Editor: Matthew Seeley

Managing Editor: Marah Bellegarde

Senior Product Manager: Debra Myette-Flis

Editorial Assistant: Samantha Zullo

Vice President, Career and Professional Marketing: Jennifer Baker

Executive Marketing Manager: Wendy Mapstone

Senior Marketing Manager: Kristin McNary

Associate Marketing Manager: Jonathan Sheehan

Production Director: Carolyn S. Miller

Content Project Manager: Thomas Heffernan

Senior Art Director: Jack Pendleton

Technology Project Manager: Patricia Allen

Library of Congress Control Number: 2010942915

ISBN-13: 978-1-435-48761-1

ISBN-10: 1-4354-8761-3

Delmar
5 Maxwell Drive
Clifton Park, NY 12065-2919
USA

Cengage Learning products are represented in Canada by Nelson Education, Ltd.

For your lifelong learning solutions, visit **delmar.cengage.com**

Visit our corporate website at **cengage.com**.

Printed in the United States of America
1 2 3 4 5 6 7 16 15 14 13 12 11

CONTENTS

TO THE LEARNER

Congratulations on choosing health care for your career! You will make a difference in so many lives. We, the authors, wish you success in your health profession.

This workbook is designed to be used in conjunction with your textbook. The question styles include fill-in-the-blank, multiple-choice, matching, diagram labeling, and short answer. In addition, we have provided questions and scenarios to stimulate critical thinking and provide discussions in areas such as ethics. These are especially interesting from the perspective that there may not be any right or wrong answers. Rather, you will need to choose actions that are appropriate for the given situations.

These thought questions are designed to also improve your oral communication skills. These skills will become increasingly important to you as your career advances. Additional activities/labs have been provided, as has information (extended concepts) that goes beyond that provided in the text.

Good luck, and have a great school year.

HOW TO USE THIS WORKBOOK

Your workbook is straightforward. Each chapter has a series of headings as follows:

Additional Questions—These questions relate to the topics found in that chapter and go beyond the questions provided in the textbook. They include multiple-choice, matching, and short answer and fill-in-the-blank questions. Labeling activities are also included.

Additional Activities/Labs—These are interesting and enlightening activities provided in the given chapter.

Extended Concepts—A simple concept from the given chapter is expanded beyond what was provided in the textbook. Some of these concepts are extremely interesting and may be about things of which you have never before heard!

What Do You Think?—These are situations or questions like those that may occur during your career. When dealing with ethical issues, you may need to make choices that are the best for given situations. (*Hint:* There may be more than one choice for each situation!) Some of these dilemmas are guaranteed to spark some lively debate among your peers.

No matter how badly you want to do well in this or any other course, you will have a hard time making the grade without good study skills. Simply stated, you need to be prepared each and every day for class. This includes reading the assigned readings, which means *really* reading the assigned readings and being able to explain both what the authors wrote and how it applies to you!

Being prepared also means completing the questions in both your textbook and workbook. These questions are included not as filler to make the book appear bigger, but, rather, to provide you with a means of seeing how well you are grasping the material.

It is also important that you participate in class discussions and reflect on what is said in class. Of course, that can happen only if you go to class!

With all of the extracurricular activities, social activities, video games, and television programs available to you, it may seem impossible to find time to study. Consider for a moment, however, what and where you want to be 10 years from now. Are you more likely to accomplish your future goals by playing video games or by studying?

Here are some basic guidelines to help you.

1. Find a place to study and turn off distractions such as your cell phone. This place must be well lit, comfortable, and quiet, with no distractions. If you have no such place where you live, perhaps you could use a library or an available room at your school.

2. Know where to get help. If you do not understand something, ask either your teacher or an expert in the field you are studying. Learn to use additional resource information in your library and on the Internet. Send for information from various organizations.

3. Share your knowledge with others, and listen to them. By teaching others what you know, you not only help them, but you also help to solidify that information in your mind. Of potentially equal importance is listening to your fellow students who may know more about a subject than do you.

4. Take good notes. Listen in class and take notes. Write down only the main points. Many students also rewrite their notes after class. This serves a twofold purpose. Not only are the resulting notes more legible, but rewriting notes also affords you review of what transpired in class. Some students also find it advantageous to outline the chapters and we encourage this practice. While it may take more time upfront, it will mean less studying time in the long run and better test results because of increased understanding of the material.

5. Prepare properly for tests. Proper review of your notes, textbook, question answers, and old tests are all important in preparing for tests. A good night's sleep is also important, as is good nutrition. Think before you write. It is usually best to follow your first instinct in choosing the best answer. Pace yourself so that you have enough time to complete your tests.

If you follow these guidelines, you will increase your chances for success. If there are times when your grades are not what you expected, remember that you tried your best.

How you conduct yourself when dealing with patients may have a profound effect on their improvement. Before beginning work in your textbook or workbook, it is important that you consider the following.

Have you ever been in a hospital as a patient? If so, were you scared? Was it the knowledge of the severity of your problem or was it the fear of the unknown that frightened you? Chances are it was your lack of knowledge that was most frightening. Did a nurse walk into your room, take your blood pressure, and leave? Would you have liked to have known your blood pressure? Were you wheeled down to X-ray only to be left in the hall for more than 45 minutes without knowing whether you were forgotten or there was simply a backup of patients? Did you have blood taken and had no idea why?

Any of these scenarios can be very confusing and frustrating for people in a new and intimidating environment. It is important to remember this when you deal with your patients. These individuals and their family members are basically in a foreign land. Their everyday routines have been disrupted, they are dealing with strangers, and they are trying to understand the new and confusing language of medical terminology: "Yes, Mr. Alvarez, as a result of the exacerbation of your wife's COPD, I have noted increased gas-trapping as displayed by her increased AP diameter and alterations of her ABGs as compared to her baseline. The X-ray reports also support this, with noted radiolucency in all fields. However, what particularly disturbs me are the patchy infiltrates in the hilar region. When was the last time she was afebrile?" Would you be able to understand this information and the question, and would it comfort you?

Although your knowledge of medical jargon will become extensive, it is imperative to consider that your patients may never have been exposed to medical terms. Make it your goal to break down complex terms and concepts so that patients truly understand what is going on. Eliminate the fear of the unknown.

When you hear the term *communication,* you probably think of written and oral forms of information transmission. The non-oral aspects of communication are very powerful, however, and therefore should never be overlooked. Being able to "read" a person's nonverbal communication is a skill you must develop if you want to be an effective communicator. Watching facial expressions, body movements and positions, and eye contact, as well as noting speaking tone, will help you to interpret a patient's level of understanding, fears, perceptions, attitudes, and so forth.

Also remember that communication is a two-way street. Your appearance and professional bearing will play a major role in how patients react to you. Something as simple as a smile can open many doors. Be relaxed. If you constantly check your watch or move toward the door, you will be signaling your patients to terminate discussion, telling them that you do not have any more time for them.

Regardless of the field you choose in health care, never lose sight of one question: "How would I want to be treated if I were in that patient's situation?" Never belittle or argue with a patient. Never play "I can top this" by telling a patient about your problems. Be sincere. If phoniness is spotted, the bridge of trust between patient and professional may never be built.

Using positive interaction skills may be trying at times. Some people are just plain difficult. In such cases, do the best you can and leave it at that. But also be aware that some people try to hide their fears or confusion behind arrogance, rage, or silence. Never lose sight of the fact that patients have given up familiar surroundings such as home, family, and friends. They have given up privacy, which can be extremely embarrassing. (Have you ever worn a hospital gown or used a bedpan?) They are now dependent on the knowledge and skills of total strangers. In many cases, their very lives are in the hands of strangers, which can be a terrifying experience.

Cultural and language barriers can also serve to block effective communication. Some of you may think that taking a foreign language is just meeting a requirement; should you choose to do so, however, you may be the only one who can communicate with an individual during an emergency situation. This ability should not be taken lightly; it may save a person's life.

Communication is the key to trust between you and your patient. Make time to develop this link. As patients open up to you, you may learn about their lifestyles, familial disease histories, or occupations, all of which may give clues to their disease processes and thus aid in developing more effective treatment regimens. A small investment of time can pay off with big dividends.

Fundamentals of Anatomy and Physiology

CHAPTER **1**

Medical Terminology: The Language of Medicine

ADDITIONAL QUESTIONS

Multiple-Choice

Circle the best answer for each of the following questions.

1. A medical term for a disease-producing organism is called:

   a. harmless

   b. pathogenic

   c. physiological

   d. inflammatory

2. The foundation of a word is its:

   a. prefix

   b. root

   c. suffix

   d. etiology

3. The medical term for inflammation of the skin is:

   a. dermatitis

   b. epidermis

   c. hypodermis

   d. paradermotomy

4. In the term *hyperglycemia,* its prefix is:

   a. *hyper*

   b. *glyc/o*

   c. *emia*

   d. *glycemia*

5. A physician who specializes in studying tissues is a (an):

   a. cytologist

   b. audiologist

   c. histologist

   d. cardiologist

6. The term for difficulty in swallowing is:

   a. dyspepsia

   b. dysphagia

   c. analgesia

   d. ectophasia

7. Something that is not indicated would be:

   a. proposed

   b. indicated

   c. hypoindicated

   d. contraindicated

8. The term *leukocytopenia* means:

   a. a normal level of blood cells

   b. an increase in red blood cells

   c. a decrease in white blood cells

   d. an increase in white blood cells

9. The medical abbreviation for the procedure to be performed on a pulseless person is:

   a. NPO

   b. CBC

   c. ASHD

   d. CPR

10. Prior to surgery, the medical abbreviation on the chart that indicates no eating or drinking is:

   a. NPR

   b. PRN

   c. CNS

   d. NPO

Matching 1

Match the following combining terms with their definitions.

____	1. *phag/o*	a.	woman
____	2. *leuk/o*	b.	blood
____	3. *hepat/o*	c.	vessel
____	4. *gynec/o*	d.	gland
____	5. *erythr/o*	e.	liver
____	6. *dermat/o*	f.	red
____	7. *angi/o*	g.	bone
____	8. *gastr/o*	h.	swallow
____	9. *oste/o*	i.	stomach
____	10. *aden/o*	j.	skin
		k.	intestine
		l.	white

Matching 2

Match the following singular and plural endings.

____	1. *-a*	a.	*-i*
____	2. *-ex, -ix*	b.	*-ices*
____	3. *-is*	c.	*-a*
____	4. *-nx*	d.	*-ae*
____	5. *-um*	e.	*-nges*
____	6. *-us*	f.	*-es*

Short Answer and Fill-in-the-Blank

1. What are endorphins?

_____

_____

_____

_____

_____

_____

2. What are some of the psychological effects of humor?

_____

_____

_____

_____

_____

_____

3. Provide the correct combining form for each of the following:

   a. _____ gland

   b. _____ tumor or mass

   c. _____ black

   d. _____ mouth

   e. _____ vein

   f. _____ pus

   g. _____ abdominal wall

   h. _____ clot

   i. _____ muscle

4. Define each of the following medical terms:

   a. immunology

   _____

   _____

   b. histology

   _____

   _____

   c. cytology

   _____

   _____

   d. thrombosis

   _____

   _____

   e. splenectomy

   _____

   _____

   f. bradycardia

   _____

   _____

   g. tracheostenosis

   _____

   _____

   h. dysphonia

   _____

   _____

5. _____ is the term for a disease-producing organism, and a (an) _____ is an individual who studies them.

6. The root word, or stem, of a medical term usually comes from the _____ or _____ language.

7. Provide the correct medical abbreviation for each of the following:

   a. acquired immune deficiency syndrome _____

   b. give twice a day _____

   c. nothing by mouth _____

   d. technique performed on someone who has apnea and no pulse _____

   e. a buildup of fluid in the heart _____

   f. when needed _____

   g. intensive care unit _____

   h. a patient says he cannot catch his breath _____

Labeling

Label the procedures in the following figure with the correct medical term.

A.
(cutting into a bone)

B.
(making a permanent
new opening in a bone)

Applied Suction
for Tapping

Catheter

C.
(surgical puncture and
tapping of a bone)

D.
(surgical repair of a
damaged bone)

E.
(removal of a bone)

A. _____   C. _____   E. _____

B. _____   D. _____

ADDITIONAL ACTIVITIES/LABS

1. After being split into groups, prepare for a spelling bee. You must not only spell the word correctly but also give the proper definition. Make sure your pronunciation is correct. Each contestant must conclude with the proper pronunciation to get full credit.

2. Either individually or in a group, develop a crossword puzzle or word search game containing fifteen medical terms.

Extended Concepts

The word *phobia* means "fear of." Human beings have many fears, and, believe it or not, most fears have medical names. For example, the fear of heights is called *acrophobia*. The fear of blood is *hemophobia*. Again, notice how knowing the term for blood (*hemo*) and the term for fear of (*phobia*) can give you the actual definition. Someone can even have a fear of developing a phobia. This, of course, would be called *phobophobia*, which is a somewhat redundant term! We can form many other terms relating to phobias; following is a list of just a few compiled for your information.

zoophobia—fear of animals
claustrophobia—fear of confinement
necrophobia—fear of corpses
panphobia—fear of everything
kakorrhaphiophobia—fear of failure
pyrophobia—fear of fire
megalophobia—fear of large objects
pharmacophobia—fear of medicine
autophobia—fear of self
microphobia—fear of small objects
ergasiophobia—fear of work

What Do You Think?

Over the past few years, you probably have heard news reports about physicians aiding in the suicides of individuals who have terminal illnesses. What are your feelings regarding "the right to die"? What are your feelings regarding physicians assisting patients to die?

CHAPTER **2**

Overview of the Human Body

ADDITIONAL QUESTIONS

Multiple-Choice

Circle the best answer for each of the following questions.

1. The term for the study of body structure is:

    a. pathology

    b. anatomy

    c. physiology

    d. cytology

2. Study of tissue structure and function:

    a. cytology

    b. dermatology

    c. histology

    d. anatomy

3. The study of the function of the body systems:

    a. physiology

    b. anatomy

    c. pathology

    d. cytology

4. What structure separates the thoracic cavity from the abdominopelvic cavity?

    a. navel

    b. diaphragm

    c. nipple

    d. liver

5. The plane dividing the body into left and right sections is called the:

   a. frontal plane

   b. median plane

   c. horizontal plane

   d. midtransverse plane

6. What is the correct ordering from simple to complex?

   a. cell, tissues, systems, organs, organism

   b. organism, systems, tissues, cells

   c. cells, tissues, organs, organisms, systems

   d. cells, tissues, organs, systems, organism

7. The gallbladder is found in which abdominal quadrant?

   a. right upper

   b. right lower

   c. left upper

   d. left lower

8. Which plane divides the body and its parts into superior and inferior portions?

   a. sagittal

   b. midsagittal

   c. cranial

   d. transverse

9. Nearest to the point of origin:

   a. distal

   b. anterior

   c. proximal

   d. superior

10. The thoracic cavity contains the following organs:

    a. lungs, heart, and stomach

    b. brain, spinal cord, and eyes

    c. heart, lungs, and esophagus

    d. stomach, spleen, and lungs

Matching 1

Match the following directional terms with their definitions.

_____ 1. superior	a. caudal
_____ 2. lateral	b. away from the point of origin
_____ 3. proximal	c. toward midline
_____ 4. distal	d. cranial
_____ 5. medial	e. away from midline
_____ 6. inferior	f. toward the point of origin

Matching 2

Match the following organs to their correct combining terms.

_____ 1. lung	a. *cardi/o*
_____ 2. liver	b. *pneum/o*
_____ 3. stomach	c. *col/o*
_____ 4. large intestine	d. *enter/o*
_____ 5. small intestine	e. *hepat/o*
_____ 6. heart	f. *gastr/o*

Short Answer and Fill-in-the-Blank

1. Your lungs take in approximately _____ quarts of air and produce approximately 1 _____ of mucus daily.

2. What are cilia?

   _____

   _____

   _____

3. Why is saliva important?

   _____

   _____

   _____

4. Where are nearly half the bones of the skeleton found?

   _____

5. Why do we compare cells to bricks?

   _____

   _____

   _____

Labeling

1. Label the body cavities illustrated in the following figure.

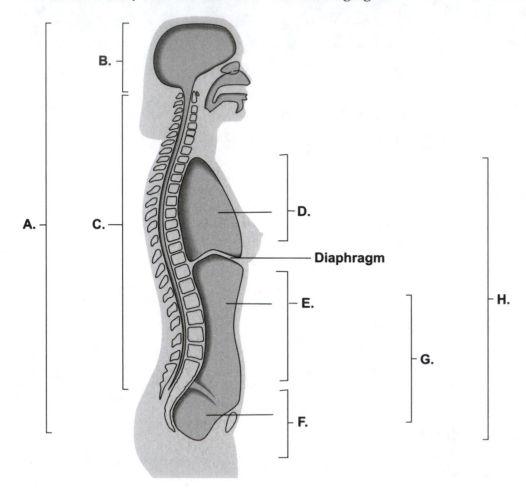

A. _____   D. _____   G. _____

B. _____   E. _____   H. _____

C. _____   F. _____

2. Label the organs located in the various cavities shown in the following figure. Include any applicable combining forms.

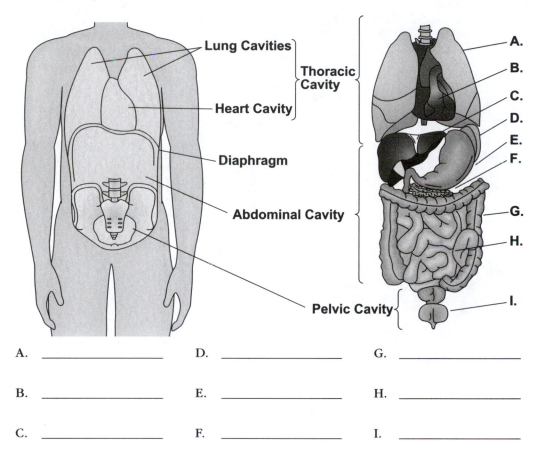

A. _____ D. _____ G. _____

B. _____ E. _____ H. _____

C. _____ F. _____ I. _____

ADDITIONAL ACTIVITIES/LABS

1. Utilizing your textbook and other resource material, make your own amazing facts of the human body booklet. Keep these facts within an organized diary.

2. Using anatomical charts or pictures of various systems, come up with sentences that utilize the following direction terms: *medial, distal, proximal, anterior, posterior, lateral, peripheral, dorsal, ventral*. Develop one sentence per directional term. For example, "The intestines are inferior to the stomach."

Extended Concepts

The term *peripheral* is used to describe location or position of the human body. Peripheral circulation is an important concept in assessing the adequacy of the pumping action of the heart and the amount of blood that is being pumped (known as *cardiac output*). Because the nail beds of both the fingers and toes are highly vascularized (i.e., they contain many blood vessels), we can determine the adequacy of perfusion by squeezing a fingernail, releasing it, and watching how it "pinks up." The blood returning to this area is what causes the nail beds to pink up. This is referred to as *reperfusion*. The more quickly a nail bed pinks up, the better the blood flow (*perfusion*). The temperature of the big toe is another way to determine adequacy of perfusion. Generally speaking, the warmer the big toe, the better the perfusion.

What Do You Think?

A baboon liver was given to a human who was dying from hepatitis B. If a human liver was used, it would have been destroyed by this disease; a baboon's liver, however, appears to be resistant to hepatitis B. Is it morally/ethically right to sacrifice animals to save humans? What about using animals for research into human diseases?

C H A P T E R **3**

The Raw Materials: Cells, Tissues, Organs, and Systems

ADDITIONAL QUESTIONS

Multiple-Choice

Circle the best answer for each of the following questions.

1. The movement of water across a semipermeable membrane is called:

    a. diffusion

    b. osmosis

    c. phagocytosis

    d. exocytosis

2. What substance in the nucleus contains the blueprint for a new cell?

    a. RNA

    b. DNA

    c. nucleolus

    d. lysosome

3. The microorganism that causes the common cold:

    a. bacterium

    b. virus

    c. fungus

    d. protozoa

4. Postural muscles, such as muscles of the neck, are in constant need of energy. Therefore, these muscle cells contain and maintain higher quantities of what type of organelles than do cells not requiring high-energy stores?

    a. mitochondria

    b. nucleus

    c. ribosomes

    d. endoplasmic reticulum

5. This part of the cell cycle is cell division.

    a. mitosis

    b. interphase

    c. cytokinesis

    d. metaphase

6. Adipose tissue is a form of:

    a. cartilage

    b. soft connective tissue

    c. epithelium

    d. cardiac tissue

7. Which muscle is voluntary?

    a. cardiac

    b. visceral

    c. skeletal

    d. nervous

8. Which system is responsible for the production of RBCs?

    a. cardiovascular

    b. skeletal

    c. endocrine

    d. respiratory

9. The lay term for the largest laryngeal cartilage is:

    a. sternum

    b. breast bone

    c. Adam's apple

    d. collar bone

10. In this phase of cellular reproduction, the chromosomes line up in the center of the cell:

    a. metaphase

    b. anaphase

    c. prophase

    d. telophase

Matching 1

Match the following cellular structures with their definitions.

____ 1. cell membrane

____ 2. nucleolus

____ 3. ribosome

____ 4. lysosome

____ 5. mitochondria

____ 6. endoplasmic reticulum

____ 7. Golgi apparatus

____ 8. centrioles

____ 9. chromatin

____ 10. cytoplasm

a. a series of transport channels in the cell, having two distinct forms

b. where RNA is synthesized

c. produces cell energy

d. digests old cells

e. contains DNA

f. gel-like substance in which the cellular organelles float

g. plays a critical role in cell division

h. composed of RNA

i. surrounds the cells and allows certain substances in and other substances out

j. puts proteins into vesicles

Matching 2

Match the following stages of cellular reproduction to their definitions.

____ 1. meiosis

____ 2. mitosis

____ 3. prophase

____ 4. metaphase

____ 5. anaphase

____ 6. telophase

a. nucleus disappears, spindle forms

b. chromosomes line up in center of cell

c. sexual reproduction

d. chromosomes pull away

e. spindle disappears, chromosomes are far apart

f. asexual reproduction

Short Answer and Fill-in-the-Blank

1. List the six common processes associated with most cells in the human body.

_____

_____

_____

_____

_____

_____

2. This is one of the smallest organisms known. It can be viewed only through an electron microscope, and it is the cause of the common cold. _____

3. This organism is smaller than bacteria; it cannot live outside its host, and it can cause typhus. _____

4. _____ and the _____ _____ are responsible for environmental control in the cell.

5. List the four main groups of tissues in the body.

_____ _____ _____ _____

Labeling 1

Label the various parts of the cell in the following figure.

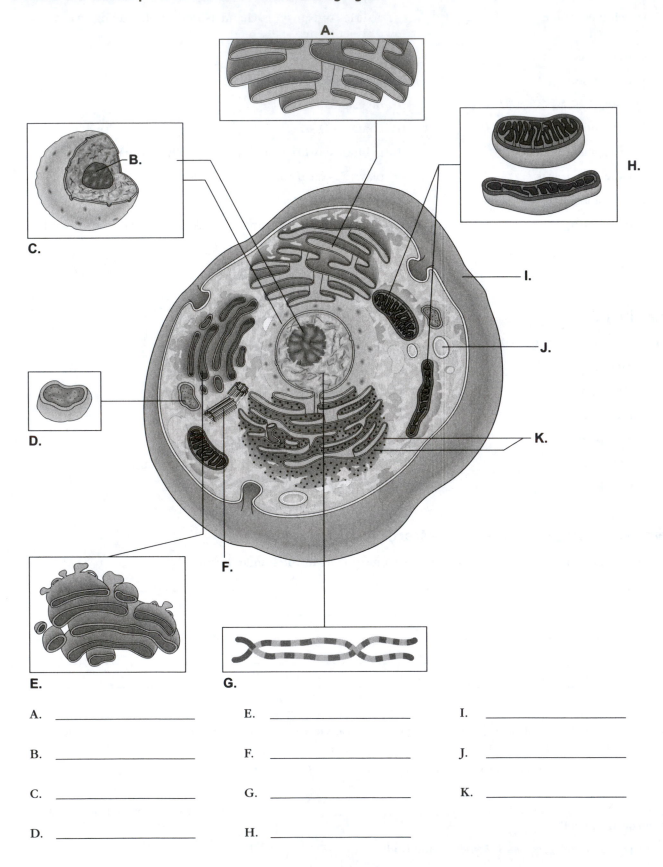

A. _____	E. _____	I. _____
B. _____	F. _____	J. _____
C. _____	G. _____	K. _____
D. _____	H. _____	

Labeling 2

Label each of the body systems in the following figures.

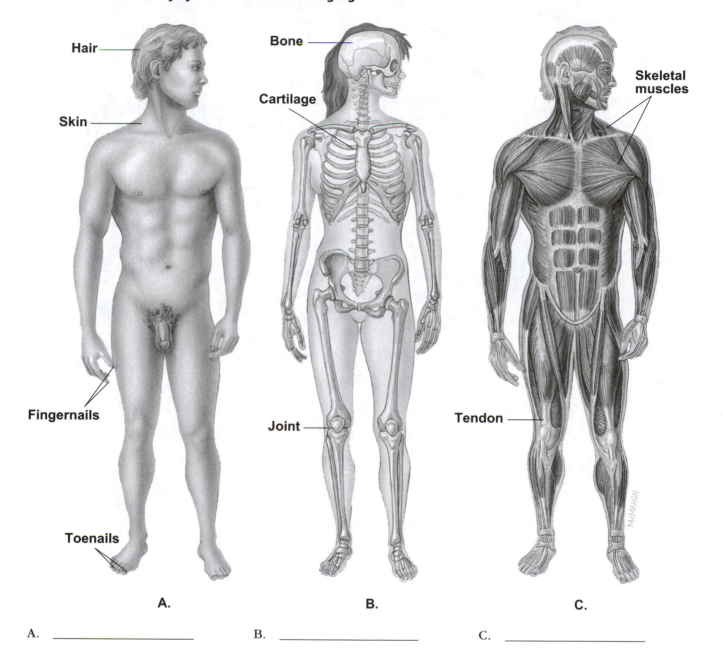

Hair

Skin

Fingernails

Toenails

Bone

Cartilage

Joint

Skeletal muscles

Tendon

A.

B.

C.

A. _____

B. _____

C. _____

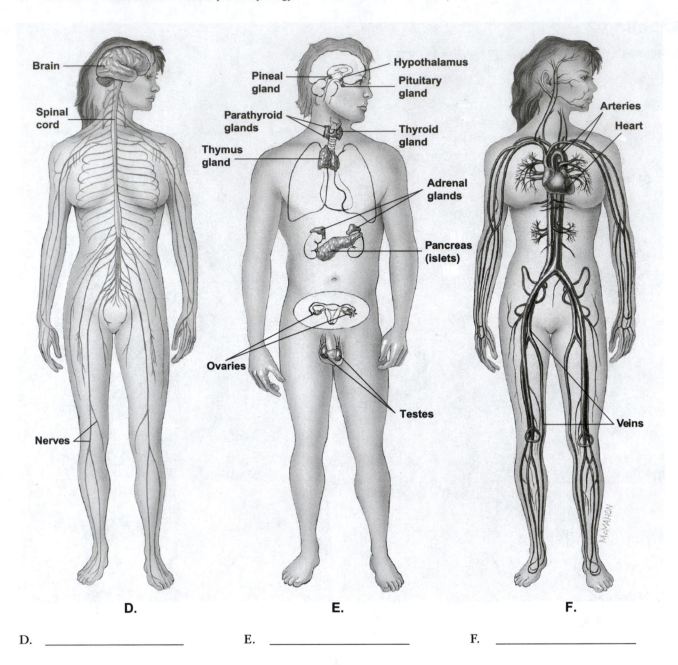

Brain

Spinal
cord

Nerves

D.

Pineal
gland

Parathyroid
glands

Thymus
gland

Ovaries

Hypothalamus

Pituitary
gland

Thyroid
gland

Adrenal
glands

Pancreas
(islets)

Testes

E.

Arteries

Heart

Veins

F.

D. _____

E. _____

F. _____

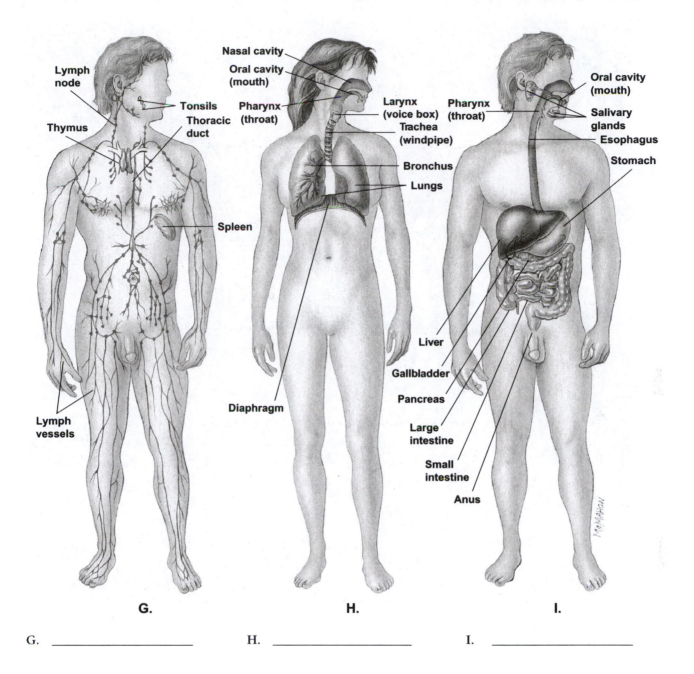

G.

H.

I.

G. _____   H. _____   I. _____

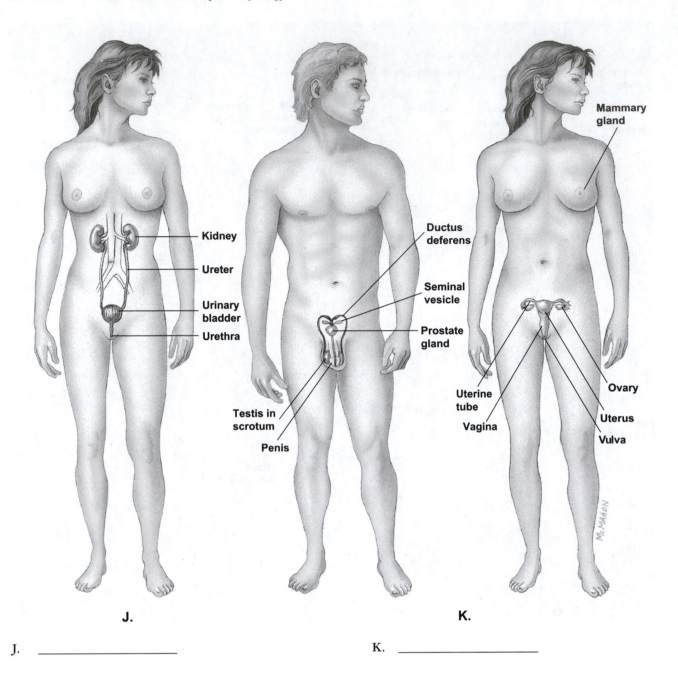

J.

K.

J. _____

K. _____

ADDITIONAL ACTIVITIES/LABS

1. Using a toothpick, gently scrape the inside of your mouth. Prepare a microscope slide from that scraping. Draw and describe your observations as you examine this slide under the microscope. Make a similar slide using two algae from a pond. List the similarities and differences between the two slides.

2. Create clay models of a cell and label the various cell parts with explanations of their functions.

Extended Concepts

Cellular Division

Somatic cells (the type of cells that compose your body tissue) multiply by the process known as *mitosis*. In mitosis, a single cell divides into two daughter cells. The process of division occurs in five stages or phases. In mitosis, the same number of chromosomes are present in each daughter cell as are present in the original cell.

However, germ cells, and our sperm and ova cells, divide by *meiosis*. These cells combine to germinate, or form a new human being. In meiosis, two successive divisions of the original cell nucleus produce half the number of chromosomes that was contained in the original somatic cell. Therefore, when the sperm from the male combines with the ova, or egg, from the female, they fuse to form a cell (called a *zygote*) having a full set of chromosomes contributed from both the male and female parents.

Ectoderm Cells, Mesoderm Cells, and Endoderm Cells

A growing fetus develops all of the necessary parts of the body from three types of cells. *Ectoderm* cells form skin, hair, nails, teeth, mammary glands, and the nervous system. *Mesoderm* cells form the skeleton, muscles, circulatory system (the veins, heart, and arteries), and the urogenital system (the sex organs, kidneys, and bladder). *Endoderm* cells form the inner linings of the digestive system and the respiratory system, and mesoderm cells create the balance of these systems.

What Do You Think?

What are your feelings regarding providing free hypodermic syringes to IV drug users as a means to stem the spread of AIDS and hepatitis B? Discuss the pros and cons of implementing such a program in your community.

CHAPTER **4**

The Integumentary System

ADDITIONAL QUESTIONS

Multiple-Choice

Circle the best answer for each of the following questions.

1. What degree of burn is a sunburn?

    a. first

    b. second

    c. third

    d. fourth

2. Which of the following layers of skin is closest to the bone?

    a. hypodermis

    b. dermis

    c. corium

    d. epidermis

3. Which of the following sweat glands secrete oil at the hair follicle?

    a. sebaceous

    b. apocrine

    c. eccrine

    d. creatine

4. Which of the following statements is true about melanin, melanocytes, and skin color?

    a. Adult humans, despite race or gender, have the same amount of melanocytes per skin square inch; skin color difference is due to the amount of melanin secreted from the standard number of melanocytes.

    b. Different skin colors and tones are due to different amounts and arrangements of melanocytes.

    c. The more melanin produced, the lighter the skin.

    d. Melanocyte absolute numbers are inversely proportional to the concentration of melanin in the skin; in other words, the more melanocytes, the less pigment can be secreted and can ultimately survive in the skin.

5. Another term for sweat gland is a (an) _____ gland.

   a. sebaceous

   b. pineal

   c. suderiferous

   d. adrenal

6. The origin of a disease is its:

   a. pathology

   b. physiology

   c. prognosis

   d. etiology

7. When signs and symptoms of a disease either partially or completely disappear, it is said to be in:

   a. acute phase

   b. remission

   c. subacute phase

   d. chronic stasis

8. The body's ability to maintain a normal state despite internal and external influences is:

   a. hemostasis

   b. vasodilation

   c. homeostasis

   d. autoregulation

9. Which of the following are true of fever?

   a. can be caused by bacterial pyrogens

   b. can cause tachypnea

   c. increases oxygen consumption

   d. all of the above

10. Hair and nails are both composed of fibrous protein called:

    a. melanin

    b. keratin

    c. cartlidge

    d. corium

Matching 1

Match the following terms with their definitions.

_____ 1. keratin   a. fat

_____ 2. lipocytes   b. cools the body

_____ 3. sebaceous   c. oil

_____ 4. suderiforous   d. true skin

_____ 5. melanin   e. found in hair and nails

_____ 6. corium   f. darkening of the skin

Matching 2

Match the following terms with their definitions.

_____ 1. dermatitis   a. black-and-blue mark

_____ 2. laceration   b. abnormal scar growth

_____ 3. urticaria   c. sunburn without blisters

_____ 4. contusion   d. tiny pinpoint purple bruise marks

_____ 5. ecchymosis   e. tissue injury that does not break open skin

_____ 6. first-degree burn   f. hives

_____ 7. cicatrix   g. a normally forming scar

_____ 8. keloid   h. blackhead

_____ 9. petechiae   i. general term for skin inflammation

_____ 10. comedo   j. jagged opening or wound of the skin

Short Answer and Fill-in-the-Blank

1. Differentiate between sebaceous and sudoriferous glands.

2. _____ is the study of the origin of a disease.

3. A(n) _____ disease is one of untraceable or unknown origin.

4. _____ is a term used to describe a stage that some diseases go into where they either partially or completely disappear.

5. List the major vital signs that are normally monitored:

_____ _____ _____ _____

Labeling 1

Label the components of the skin in the following figure.

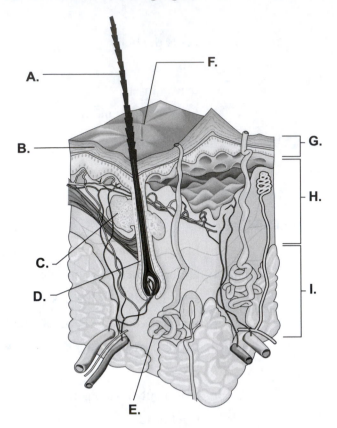

A. _____   D. _____   G. _____

B. _____   E. _____   H. _____

C. _____   F. _____   I. _____

Labeling 2

Label the skin lesions in the following figure.

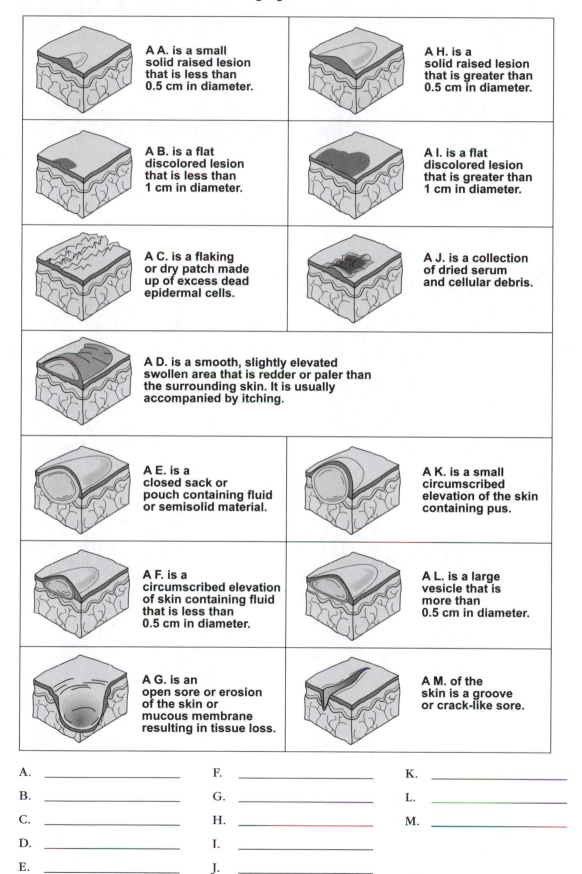

A A. is a small
solid raised lesion
that is less than
0.5 cm in diameter.

A H. is a
solid raised lesion
that is greater than
0.5 cm in diameter.

A B. is a flat
discolored lesion
that is less than
1 cm in diameter.

A I. is a flat
discolored lesion
that is greater than
1 cm in diameter.

A C. is a flaking
or dry patch made
up of excess dead
epidermal cells.

A J. is a collection
of dried serum
and cellular debris.

A D. is a smooth, slightly elevated
swollen area that is redder or paler than
the surrounding skin. It is usually
accompanied by itching.

A E. is a
closed sack or
pouch containing fluid
or semisolid material.

A K. is a small
circumscribed
elevation of the skin
containing pus.

A F. is a
circumscribed elevation
of skin containing fluid
that is less than
0.5 cm in diameter.

A L. is a large
vesicle that is
more than
0.5 cm in diameter.

A G. is an
open sore or erosion
of the skin or
mucous membrane
resulting in tissue loss.

A M. of the
skin is a groove
or crack-like sore.

A. _____

B. _____

C. _____

D. _____

E. _____

F. _____

G. _____

H. _____

I. _____

J. _____

K. _____

L. _____

M. _____

ADDITIONAL ACTIVITIES/LABS

Using a number of resources (perhaps including input from a dermatologist), develop a wellness pamphlet for the care of your skin. If done well, provide copies to the school.

Extended Concepts

Plastic surgery, also known as reconstructive surgery, involves correcting deformities that result from birth defects, disease processes, or injuries. For example, burn victims can receive skin grafts to replace destroyed tissue. A section of skin having living cells is taken from a compatible donor and attached to the damaged area on the recipient. *Xenografts* are skin grafts from incompatible donors. Xenografts will eventually be rejected, but they do provide time for the recipient's tissue to heal.

What Do You Think?

A 60-year-old patient is dying from a disease for which there is no known cure. Death may come tomorrow or within three years. Three weeks ago the patient slipped into a coma. There is no response to verbal commands and no reflex responses. Feeding via tubes placed in the stomach is the only way nourishment can be provided. The patient has minimal health insurance, and the family is poor. Discuss in class the option of withholding feeding to let the patient die. Is this an ethical option? Is this a legal option? What would you do?

C H A P T E R **5**

The Skeletal System

ADDITIONAL QUESTIONS

Multiple-Choice

Circle the best answer for each of the following questions.

1. The bone cells that build new bone are:

   a. osteoclasts

   b. osteocytes

   c. osteoblasts

   d. osteofibroids

2. Which kind of fracture breaks through the skin?

   a. simple

   b. closed

   c. compound

   d. greenstrick

3. Rickets can be a result of a deficiency in:

   a. iron

   b. vitamin B_{12}

   c. vitamin D

   d. phosphorus

4. The phalanges and ulna are examples of what type of bone?

   a. irregularly shaped

   b. long

   c. short

   d. flat

5. The expanded ends of long bone are called:

    a. epimysia

    b. epicondyles

    c. epiphysis

    d. epiosteum

6. What type of bony tissue makes up the adult diaphysis?

    a. cancellous bone

    b. spongy bone

    c. cartilage

    d. compact bone

7. Connective tissue that attaches bone to bone:

    a. ligament

    b. cartilage

    c. tendon

    d. fascia

8. The vertebral column has how many vertebrae in the cervical, thoracic, and lumbar regions?

    a. 7, 12, 5

    b. 12, 5, 5

    c. 5, 7, 5

    d. 7, 5, 12

9. Which of the following diseases produces a humpback?

    a. lordosis

    b. kyphosis

    c. scoliosis

    d. osteosis

Matching 1

Match the following terms with their definitions.

_____ 1. tailbone   a. carpals

_____ 2. shoulder blade   b. sternum

_____ 3. upper arm bone   c. scapula

_____ 4. toes   d. radius

_____ 5. thigh bone   e. femur

_____ 6. lower leg bone   f. coccyx

_____ 7. forearm bone   g. fibula

_____ 8. wrist bones   h. tarsals

_____ 9. ankle bones   i. phalanges

_____ 10. breastbone   j. humerus

Matching 2

Match the following terms with their definitions.

_____ 1. fibrous   a. neck and forearm

_____ 2. synovial   b. found in the wrist and ankle

_____ 3. ball and socket   c. hips and shoulder

_____ 4. gliding   d. knees and elbow

_____ 5. hinge   e. found on the cranium; sutures

_____ 6. pivot   f. fluid in a joint cavity

Short Answer and Fill-in-the-Blank

1. A _____ _____ is a type of fracture that can occur without any trauma.

2. How do we know that Neanderthal humans squatted instead of sat?

   _____

   _____

   _____

3. Why is it important for the periosteum to have blood vessels, lymph vessels, and nerves?

   _____

   _____

   _____

4. There are approximately _____ _____ RBCs circulating in your blood system, and you make _____ _____ new RBCs every second.

5. _____ is a bone disease that can cause bow legs and is a result of childhood deficiencies of calcium and vitamin D.

Labeling 1

Label the various components of the skeletal system in the following figure.

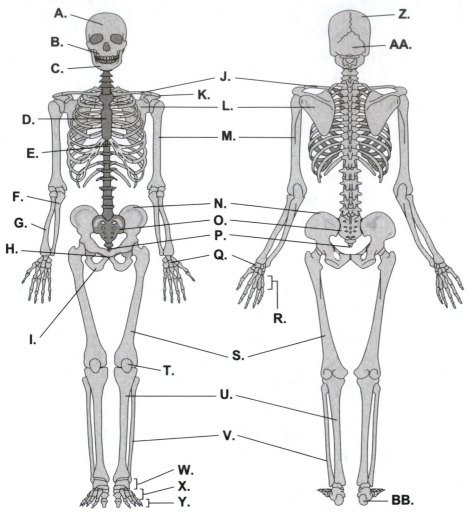

A. _____   K. _____   U. _____

B. _____   L. _____   V. _____

C. _____   M. _____   W. _____

D. _____   N. _____   X. _____

E. _____   O. _____   Y. _____

F. _____   P. _____   Z. _____

G. _____   Q. _____   AA. _____

H. _____   R. _____   BB. _____

I. _____   S. _____

J. _____   T. _____

Labeling 2

Label the main parts of the long bone in the following figure.

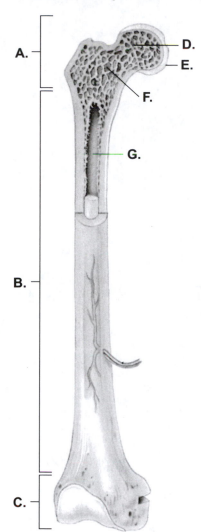

A. _____

B. _____

C. _____

D. _____

E. _____

F. _____

G. _____

Labeling 3

Label the various parts of the knee joint and surrounding structures.

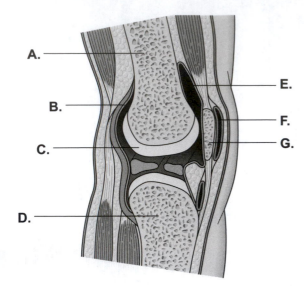

A. _____

B. _____

C. _____

D. _____

E. _____

F. _____

G. _____

ADDITIONAL ACTIVITIES/LABS

1. Referring to pictures in your textbook and using white paper, scissors, and glue, create your own life-size skeleton. You can also have an individual lie down on a large piece of paper and trace the person's outline to give the overall shape and size from which to begin your work.

2. Bring in or describe various "real-life" devices that mimic the pivot, fibrous, ball-and-socket, and hinge joints.

Extended Concepts

More on Bone Diseases

There are many causes of bone disease. Metabolic disorders of the body can lead to insufficient storage of vital minerals such as calcium and phosphorus. Bones can also be weakened by kidney diseases that cause an imbalance of those minerals within the body. Nutrition plays a key role in bone health. Rickets in children (osteomalacia in adults) is caused by insufficient levels of vitamin D. In addition, the lack of vitamin C can affect bone tissue and result in the disease *scurvy*. This disease was quite common in our distant past when sailors would take long voyages and not have fresh fruit to supply the needed vitamin C. This is the source of a famous nickname. British sailors took limes on board ship to prevent scurvy; hence, they were known as "limies." This is also the source of the famous line from pirate movies: "Avast, yee scurvy dogs."

Bone disease can also result from ingestion of materials in the environment. A classic example is women who painted radium on clock dials to make them glow in the dark. They often licked the small paint brushes to form a tip. As a result, they ingested radium, a radioactive material. Many died from anemia or bone cancer.

What Do You Think?

Intubation is the technique of placing a hollow plastic tube into a person's airway either to allow the individual to breathe easier on his or her own or to allow assisted breathing by another person or a machine. Intubation mannequins can be used to practice this technique; however, intubating a mannequin is not quite the same as intubating a human. It is important to note that the more you practice, the better you get at this procedure, and the better you are, the less damage you are likely to cause your patient. Efficiency in intubation may make a difference in the individual's survivability.

Mr. Robinson, a patient at the hospital where you work, has gone into cardiac arrest. He was intubated and cardiopulmonary resuscitation (CPR) was begun. Despite the heroic efforts of the doctors and health care professionals, he could not be revived. Given that he is dead and already intubated, is there anything wrong with removing the tube and quickly practicing a few intubations before his family is allowed to view his body?

CHAPTER **6**

The Muscular System

ADDITIONAL QUESTIONS

Multiple-Choice

Circle the best answer for each of the following questions.

1. The fibrous tissue that attaches skeletal muscle to bone:

   a. ligaments

   b. tendons

   c. cords

   d. bursa

2. Muscles that cause movement are known as:

   a. antagonists

   b. synergists

   c. protagonists

   d. agonists

3. Which of the following is a group of anterior thigh muscles?

   a. hamstrings

   b. quadriceps

   c. peroneals

   d. gluteals

4. Which of the following is a group of buttocks muscles?

   a. psoas

   b. gluteal

   c. hamstrings

   d. quadriceps

5. Which of the following is a muscle of the lower leg?

   a. gastrocnemius

   b. latissimus dorsi

   c. deltoid

   d. hamstring

6. Muscles that are used for duration or high-endurance activity will look:

   a. white due to the excess oxygen and fat stored for energy

   b. white due to the lack of blood supply

   c. dark due to the rich blood supply to carry needed oxygen

   d. dark due to chronic tears and scar tissue in the muscle fibers

7. After death, when the body becomes stiff due to unreleased muscle contraction, the condition is referred to as:

   a. rigor mortis

   b. tetanus

   c. myalgia

   d. paralysis

8. The lack of muscle use can lead to:

   a. hypertrophy

   b. atrophy

   c. ataxia

   d. dystrophy

9. The stored carbohydrate in a muscle is called:

   a. glucose

   b. glucagon

   c. glycogen

   d. calcium

10. Which is true of the diaphragm?

    a. smooth muscle

    b. voluntary

    c. skeletal

    d. both b and c

Matching 1

Match the following terms with their definitions.

_____ 1. flexion   a. prime mover

_____ 2. rotation   b. lengthens upon movement or contraction of prime mover

_____ 3. abduction   c. movement away from midline

_____ 4. extension   d. movement toward midline

_____ 5. adduction   e. movement decreasing angle of the joint

_____ 6. antagonist   f. movement increasing angle of the joint

_____ 7. agonist   g. movement around a center axis

Matching 2

Match the following terms with their definitions.

_____ 1. myalgia

_____ 2. hernia

_____ 3. ataxia

_____ 4. cramp or spasm

_____ 5. paralysis

_____ 6. myasthenia gravis

_____ 7. Guillain-Barré syndrome

_____ 8. tendonitis

_____ 9. atrophy

_____ 10. muscular dystrophy

a. irregular muscle action; lack of coordination

b. involuntary, sudden, and violent contractions

c. partial or total loss of ability of voluntary muscles to move

d. a PNS disorder resulting in flaccid paralysis

e. a disorder in which patients experience progressive yet gradual muscle weakness

f. inherited muscle disease in which muscle fibers degenerate

g. the process of muscle wasting away; could be due to lack of nutrition, disease, or disuse

h. tenderness and pain in muscle

i. a tear in a muscle wall through which an organ protrudes

j. inflammatory condition of structure that connects muscle to bone

Short Answer and Fill-in-the-Blank

1. Muscles that cause movement are known as _____.

2. _____ is the term to describe circular motion around an axis.

3. Cardiac muscle fibers are connected to each other by _____ _____.

4. Can scar tissue effectively contract if it is located in heart muscle? _____

5. Special smooth muscles form a donut-shaped structure in the digestive system called the _____.

6. What causes wheezing during an asthma attack?

   _____

   _____

   _____

   _____

   _____

7. _____ is the term used to describe the partial contraction of a muscle with a resistance to stretching.

8. _____ is the wasting away of muscle due to lack of use.

9. _____ is a stored carbohydrate found in muscle.

10. Why are the muscles in the legs of a long-distance runner darker than those found in the hand of a quadriplegic?

   _____

   _____

   _____

   _____

   _____

Labeling 1

Label the superficial muscles of the body (anterior view).

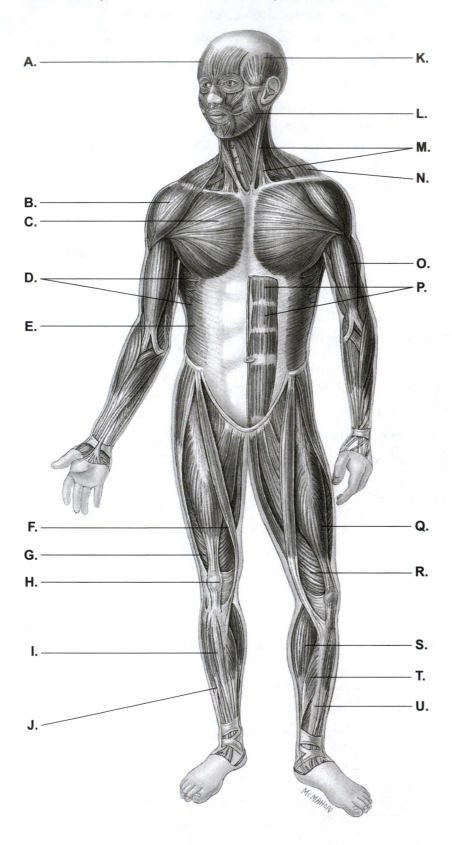

A. _____

B. _____

C. _____

D. _____

E. _____

F. _____

G. _____

H. _____

I. _____

J. _____

K. _____

L. _____

M. _____

N. _____

O. _____

P. _____

Q. _____

R. _____

S. _____

T. _____

U. _____

Labeling 2

Label the superficial muscles of the body (posterior view).

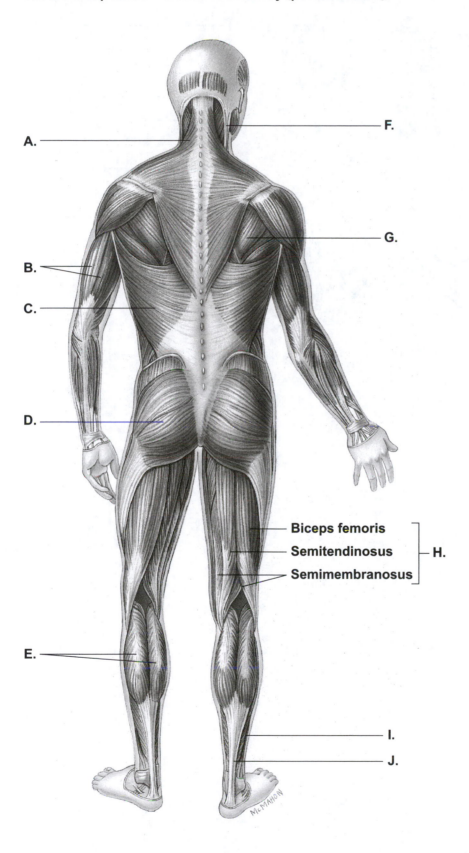

A. _____

B. _____

C. _____

D. _____

E. _____

F. _____

G. _____

H. _____

I. _____

J. _____

A.

B.

C.

D.

E.

F.

G.

Biceps femoris

Semitendinosus — H.

Semimembranosus

I.

J.

Labeling 3

Identify the various joint movements in the following figure.

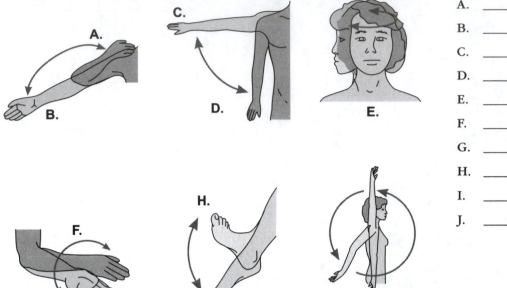

A. _____

B. _____

C. _____

D. _____

E. _____

F. _____

G. _____

H. _____

I. _____

J. _____

ADDITIONAL ACTIVITIES/LABS

After the class is divided into three groups, use resource material (obtained from the library or organizations such as the American Heart Association and Ross Laboratories) to develop wellness programs for different age groups. A wellness program should include at least a healthy diet, an exercise program, and ways to prevent or stop unhealthy habits such as excessive alcohol consumption. Group one should gear its wellness program to children and teens, group two to young to middle-age adults, and group three to older adults.

Extended Concepts

Exercise is not just for the young. As the body ages, exercise becomes even more important for a number of reasons. Exercise can help fight cardiovascular disease (including high blood pressure, heart disease, and high cholesterol). Exercise also helps maintain muscle mass, which usually decreases with age.

With age, the capacity for physical activity normally decreases. Regular exercise can actually slow that decrease by as much as 50 percent.

Regardless of age, it appears that the major cause of obesity is lack of appropriate and regular physical activity. Even after a desired amount of weight is lost, an exercise program lasting 20 minutes a day and done 3 days a week is required to keep the weight off—assuming that a proper diet is maintained.

What Do You Think?

What do you think it would be like to be confined to a wheelchair? What obstacles would this present? What if you did not have adequate bladder control?

C H A P T E R **7**

The Nervous System

ADDITIONAL QUESTIONS

Multiple-Choice

Circle the best answer for each of the following questions.

1. The following are neurotransmitter substances EXCEPT:

    a. epinephrine

    b. NE

    c. ACh

    d. cholesterol

2. What two structures make up the entire central nervous system?

    a. spinal cord and spinal nerve

    b. gray and white matter

    c. brain and spinal cord

    d. brachial and lumbar plexi

3. Choose the correct order of the CNS's protective membrane from innermost to outermost layer.

    a. pia mater, dura mater, arachnoid

    b. archnoid, dura mater, pia mater

    c. pia mater, arachoid, dura mater

    d. dura mater, arachnoid, pia mater

4. Severe damage to the spinal cord at the lumbar level may result in:

    a. quadriplegia

    b. blindness

    c. bipedalism

    d. paraplegia

5. The combination of axon terminal and receiving muscle cell is called the:

   a. node of ranvier

   b. dendrite

   c. neuromuscular junction

   d. cordae tendinae

6. Which of the following neurotransmitters can be found in the CNS, PNS, and mainly at skeletal neuromuscular synapses?

   a. norepinephrine

   b. acetylcholine

   c. epinephrine

   d. serotonin

7. Which of the following systems controls smooth muscle, cardiac muscle, and glands?

   a. somatic nervous system

   b. sensory system

   c. autonomic nervous system

   d. all of the above

8. Folds in the brain that allow for more storage of information are called:

   a. gyri

   b. sulci

   c. cortex

   d. callosum

9. Which lobe is responsible for voluntary muscle control and speech?

   a. occipital

   b. parietal

   c. temporal

   d. frontal

10. Which lobe is responsible for interpreting sound?

    a. occipital

    b. parietal

    c. temporal

    d. frontal

Matching 1

Match the following terms with their definitions.

_____ 1. meningitis

_____ 2. encephalitis

_____ 3. stroke (CVA)

_____ 4. emboli

_____ 5. hemiplegia

_____ 6. quadraplegia

_____ 7. aphasia

a. paralysis of four limbs

b. disruption of blood flow to the brain

c. inflammation of the brain

d. loss of abilty to speak or effectively communicate

e. inflammation of the protective covering of the brain and spinal cord

f. a traveling blood clot

g. paralysis on one side of the body

Matching 2

Match the following terms with their definitions.

_____ 1. medulla oblongata

_____ 2. parietal lobes

_____ 3. hypothalamus

_____ 4. motor cortex

_____ 5. frontal lobe

_____ 6. cerebellum

_____ 7. corpus callosum

_____ 8. temporal lobe

_____ 9. sulci

_____ 10. occipital lobes

a. primary area for sensory information (pain, pressure, etc.)

b. connect left and right hemispheres

c. primary area for hearing function

d. primary area (lobe) for motor function

e. fissures or furrows on the brain surface

f. primary area for vision functions

g. coordination

h. controls voluntary skeletal muscle movements

i. part of brain stem that regulates heart rate, blood pressure, respiration

j. regulate hormonal release and body temperature

Short Answer and Fill-in-the-Blank

1. In general, the nervous system is responsible for _____ _____ and for _____ and _____.

2. Another name for a efferent neuron is a _____ neuron.

3. _____ neurons carry signals from one neuron to another.

4. _____ cells provide support to neurons.

Labeling 1

Indicate the divisions of the nervous system by completing the following figure.

```
            Nervous
            System

      A.              B.

                C.          D.

                      E.          F.
```

A. _____

B. _____

C. _____

D. _____

E. _____

F. _____

Labeling 2

Label the various areas of the brain in the following figure.

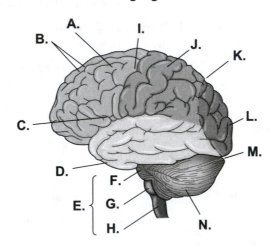

A. _____ F. _____ K. _____

B. _____ G. _____ L. _____

C. _____ H. _____ M. _____

D. _____ I. _____ N. _____

E. _____ J. _____

Labeling 3

Label the following figure of the neurons.

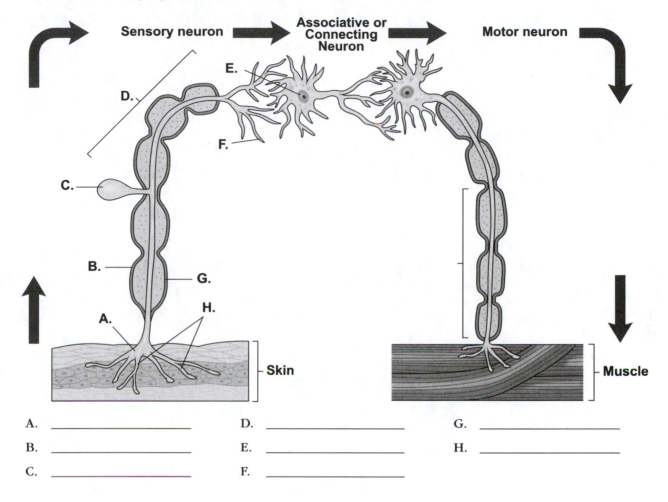

A. _____ D. _____ G. _____

B. _____ E. _____ H. _____

C. _____ F. _____

ADDITIONAL ACTIVITIES/LABS

1. Investigate the concepts of acupuncture and reflexology as they relate to the nervous system.

2. After you are assigned a nerve, tell its point of origin, whether it is sensory or motor, and what it innervates (connects).

Extended Concepts

At one time or another in our lives, we have all had to deal with pain. The pain may have resulted from athletic activities during which muscles were strained or perhaps sprained, toothaches, injuries, illness, infections, or other causes.

Pain is a symptom that something may not be right and, thus, should not be ignored. The source of the pain should be found. When the source is found, the pain can be dealt with as its cause is treated. This can be done through the use of *analgesics*. Analgesics are substances, or sometimes modalities, that can reduce the perception of pain. This can sometimes be a double-edged sword because analgesics may also affect the perception of other stimuli that are needed for normal functioning.

Examples of common analgesics used to treat mild pain are aspirin (acetylsalicylic acid) and acetaminophen (the active ingredient in Tylenol). If you have had a cavity filled, chances are that your dentist gave you an injection of novocaine to deaden the area around the tooth. This is an example of a local anesthetic used to block pain.

As the level of pain increases, the strength of the analgesic also must increase. Narcotic analgesics such as codeine and morphine are often used in such circumstances. Narcotic analgesics, however, can have serious side effects and can adversely affect the senses.

There has been increased interest in nondrug analgesic modalities such as acupuncture, electrical stimulation, biofeedback, and hypnosis. Acupuncture is the technique whereby fine needles are inserted at specific points on the body to reduce or eliminate pain. Biofeedback uses the patient's mind to control pain via relaxation and concentration. Mild electrical stimulation of certain muscles or specific nerves serves as a pain blocker.

What Do You Think?

How do you feel about nontraditional medical practices? Remember, what is nontraditional to one person may be traditional to another. Many techniques, drugs, and home remedies used in the past have been proven to be beneficial. Some, however, are dangerous or have harmful side effects. How would you choose what is right for you?

CHAPTER **8**

The Endocrine System

ADDITIONAL QUESTIONS

Multiple-Choice

Circle the best answer for each of the following questions.

1. This substance limits the excretion of urine from the body:

   a. somatotropic hormone

   b. MSH

   c. ADH

   d. ACTH

2. Hypertrophy of this gland causes goiter:

   a. pineal

   b. thyroid

   c. adrenal

   d. pituitary

3. What is the target organ for glucagon?

   a. pancreas

   b. kidneys

   c. adrenals

   d. liver

4. How do hormones and neurotransmitters (NTs) differ?

   a. Hormones are secreted by exocrine glands, and NTs are secreted from endocrine glands.

   b. Hormones are fast to take action, and NTs are slow to take effect.

   c. Hormones are secreted by endocrine glands, and NTs are released from axon terminals.

   d. b and c

5. Where are the adrenal glands located?

   a. above the kidneys

   b. in the brain stem

   c. in the chest

   d. in the neck

6. On which feedback mechanism does insulin operate?

   a. positive

   b. negative

   c. neutral

   d. neural

7. The pancreas is located in the:

   a. abdomen

   b. brain

   c. neck

   d. pelvis

8. What is the target organ for ACTH?

   a. adrenals

   b. adenoids

   c. anterior pituitary

   d. arterial walls

9. Glucagon converts what substance into glucose in times of need?

   a. insulin

   b. glycogen

   c. thymosin

   d. calcitonin

10. Polyuria (increased urination) is a symptom of:

    a. Addison disease

    b. diabetes mellitus

    c. Cushing disease

    d. Hashimoto disease

Matching 1

Match the following terms with their definitions.

_____ 1. parathyroid hormone

_____ 2. estrogen

_____ 3. testosterone

_____ 4. aldosterone

_____ 5. cortisol

_____ 6. calcitonin

_____ 7. insulin

_____ 8. epinephrine

_____ 9. melatonin

a. aids in food metabolism during stress

b. development of breasts and regulating menstruation

c. decreases blood calcium

d. allows for glucose metabolism

e. regulates secondary sexual characteristics of deep voice and facial hair

f. increases blood calcium

g. prolongs fight-or-flight response

h. influences sleep

i. controls levels of sodium and potassium

Matching 2

Match the following terms with their definitions.

_____ 1. acromegaly

_____ 2. Addison

_____ 3. diabetes mellitus

_____ 4. dwarfism

_____ 5. bone deterioration

_____ 6. testicular shrinkage

_____ 7. Graves' disease

a. steroid abuse

b. pituitary malfunction leading to enlarged hands and feet

c. decreased secretion of insulin by pancreas

d. hyperthyroidism; bulging eyes

e. hypersecretion of parathyroid hormone

f. hypofunction of adrenal gland leading to decreased immune function

g. decreased growth hormone during childhood

Short Answer and Fill-in-the-Blank

1. List the seven important glands (or groups of glands) within the body.

_____

_____

_____

_____

_____

2. What is MSH, and what is its purpose?

_____

_____

_____

_____

_____

3. _____ is the name given to the strip of tissue that connects the two large lobes of the thyroid gland.

4. _____ is the hormone that regulates the production of heat and energy in the body.

5. What are the common signs and symptoms of Graves' disease?

   _____

   _____

   _____

   _____

   _____

   _____

6. What is PTH, and what is its purpose?

   _____

   _____

   _____

   _____

   _____

   _____

7. When considering diabetes, what does **CAUTION** stand for?

   _____

   _____

   _____

   _____

   _____

Labeling

Label the glands in the following figure.

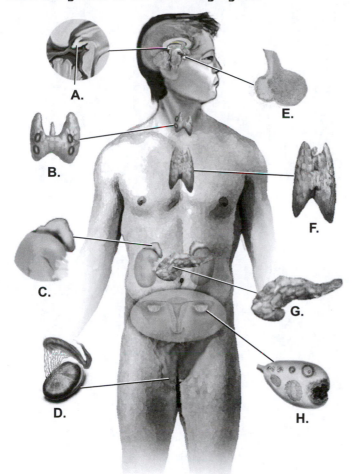

A. _____

B. _____

C. _____

D. _____

E. _____

F. _____

G. _____

H. _____

ADDITIONAL ACTIVITIES/LABS

After your teacher has assigned you an endocrine gland, make a chart that includes:

- a picture showing the gland and its location in the body

- a general description of the purpose of the gland

- a list of the gland's secretions and the functions they serve

- a list of diseases caused by over- or underproduction of these secretions

Extended Concepts

There are situations involving the endocrine system that lead to *abnormal growth*. As you already know, the pituitary gland produces the growth hormone. Too much or too little of this hormone will affect growth.

The Ellis-van Creveld syndrome is a condition wherein there is inadequate growth of the long bones during childhood. This is also known as *dwarfism*. Another form of dwarfism involves inadequate growth of the vertebrae.

Conversely, Engelmann's disease (also known as *diaphysial dysplasia*) leads to excessive growth of the long bones during childhood. This condition is commonly known as *giantism*. Individuals having giantism can reach heights of 7 to 8 feet! If this condition occurs in adults after their long bones have matured (and thus will not grow any larger), the facial bones, hands, and feet increase in size. This condition is called *acromegaly*.

Interestingly, if a tadpole has its thyroid gland removed, it never develops into a frog. In humans, if there is a deficiency in the production of thyroxine (from the thyroid gland), bone growth slows, which can lead to *cretinism*. Cretinism affects physical growth and also results in arrested mental development.

What Do You Think?

Recently, it has been postulated that the female ovaries from aborted fetuses could be implanted into infertile women to enable these women to have children. The women were infertile for a number of reasons. They may not have been able to produce eggs of their own or may have had abnormal eggs as a result of disease. The procedure has been successfully done in mice, and it is felt that humans will be next. What do you think about this possibility? What ethical issues are raised by this possibility? What rights would the mother of the fetus have if a child were born to an infertile woman using an egg from the fetus's mother's ovary?

CHAPTER **9**

The Special Senses

ADDITIONAL QUESTIONS

Multiple-Choice

Circle the best answer for each of the following questions.

1. These structures provide color vision:

   a. rods

   b. iris

   c. cones

   d. kodachrome

2. The structure responsible for balance is/are:

   a. Eustachian tubes

   b. stapes

   c. incus

   d. labyrinth

3. Which of the following correctly describes *phantom* pain?

   a. pain at the location where a vital organ was recently removed

   b. pain that originates in one part of the body but is felt in another

   c. pain that is mysteriously felt in the daytime but is elusive at nighttime

   d. pain felt in a limb that was amputated

4. Umami is (are):

   a. ringing in the ears

   b. shadows in the visual spectrum

   c. sporadic deafness and loss of equilibrium

   d. the taste of glutamates

5. Which of the following is true about the rods and cones?

   a. There are far more rods than cones.

   b. There are far more cones that rods.

   c. There are equal amounts of rods and cones.

   d. The number of rods and cones are correctable with prescription eyeglasses.

6. What is the primary function of the ossicles?

   a. amplification of the sound waves that enter the middle ear

   b. channeling of the sound waves that enter the outer ear

   c. interpretation of sound waves that enter the inner ear

   d. to vibrate the ear drum

7. Senses such as thirst, nausea, and the need to defecate are what kind of senses?

   a. special

   b. cutaneous

   c. systemic

   d. general

8. Where is the eardrum located?

   a. between the middle and inner ear

   b. between the middle and outer ear

   c. between the outer ear and labyrinth

   d. at the outer rim of the external auditory meatus

9. Arrange the ossicles in the direction that sound waves would travel through them:

   a. malleus, incus, stapes

   b. hammer, anvil, incus

   c. stirrup, anvil, hammer

   d. incus, malleus, stirrup

10. Which of the three layers of the eyeball is highly vascularized and also contains the iris?

    a. cornea

    b. choroid

    c. retina

    d. sclera

11. When there is low light, the iris will:

    a. defer activity to the rods

    b. tighten

    c. relax

    d. rely on the cones

Matching 1

Match the following terms with their definitions.

_____ 1. myopia

_____ 2. labyrinthitis

_____ 3. tinnitus

_____ 4. conjunctivitis

_____ 5. otitis media

_____ 6. amblyopia

_____ 7. Meniere's disease

_____ 8. cataracts

_____ 9. glaucoma

_____ 10. hyperopia

a. lazy eye

b. inflammation of the lining of the eye

c. a ringing sound in the ears

d. inflammation of the inner ear

e. near-sightedness

f. loss of taste

g. far-sightedness

h. chronic condition leading to progressive hearing loss and vertigo

i. infection of the middle ear

j. increased pressure in the fluid of the eye

k. clouded lens of the eye

Matching 2

Match the following terms with their definitions.

_____ 1. rods

_____ 2. cornea

_____ 3. cones

_____ 4. sclera

_____ 5. lens

_____ 6. pupil

_____ 7. lacrimal

_____ 8. vitreous

_____ 9. iris

_____ 10. aqueous

a. gland that secretes tears

b. humor that bathes the iris, pupil, and lens

c. bends light; surrounded by involuntary muscles

d. clinical term for the entire middle layer of the eyeball

e. sphincter that controls how much light passes into the eye

f. humor that occupies the posterior cavity of the eyeball

g. photoreceptor active in dim light

h. hole or circular opening in the middle of the sphincter muscle of the eyes

i. whites of the eye

j. photoreceptor active in bright light

k. transparent structure allowing outside light rays into the eye

Short Answer and Fill-in-the-Blank

1. Differentiate between the cutaneous senses and the visceral senses.

_____

_____

_____

_____

_____

2. With regard to the eye, a _____ is a substance that causes a chemical change when exposed to light.

3. What are the purposes of tears?

4. _____ _____ are needed to allow for the equalization of pressures between either side of the eardrum.

5. _____ _____ is another name for touch receptor.

6. Why is pain an important sensation?

_____

_____

_____

_____

_____

Labeling 1

Label the structures of the eye in the following figure.

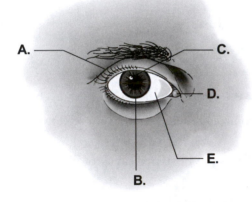

A. _____

B. _____

C. _____

D. _____

E. _____

Labeling 2

Label the structures and regions of the ear in the following figure.

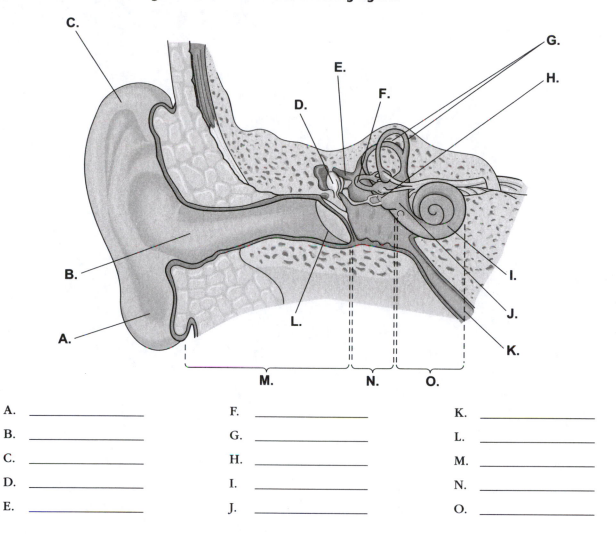

A. _____	F. _____	K. _____
B. _____	G. _____	L. _____
C. _____	H. _____	M. _____
D. _____	I. _____	N. _____
E. _____	J. _____	O. _____

ADDITIONAL ACTIVITIES/LABS

After your class has been divided into four groups, you will engage in activities to gain an appreciation for your senses. Students in group one will be blindfolded for an entire day at school; students in group two will assist those in group one with their daily functions; and the two groups will switch roles the next day. Students in group three will wear ear plugs for an entire day, and students in group four will wear nose clips for an entire day. You will then write a short essay describing how the loss of a sense affected you. Following will be a class discussion of your and your classmates' findings.

Extended Concepts

Equilibrium

Without realizing it, we are constantly influenced by gravity. If we could not negotiate gravity, we would be falling down all of the time. Fortunately, the body has three interactive systems that provide balance to allow it to function in a world with gravity. These three systems are the vestibular system, which is composed of the organs of the inner ear; vision, which gives us the sense of the horizon; and proprioception, which is the term for the body's knowledge of the position of the body parts without the assistance of the external senses (as when scratching an itchy ear in the dark).

These interrelated systems are integrated in a region near the inner ear and the cerebellum. If one system fails, you may still be able to keep your balance, as in the situation of a person who is blind being able to walk, dance, and so forth. A problem with the vestibular system, however, may affect your ability to walk. Such a problem can result from a bacterial or viral infection, certain prescription drugs, alcohol consumption, or head trauma.

What Do You Think?

A patient suffers from a condition that produces extremely foul-smelling stools. Two nurse aides who had bathed the patient were joking in the hall about needing a chainsaw to cut through the smell to get to the patient. Unfortunately the patient's family was coming down the hall to visit and overheard the remarks. Suppose you are the floor supervisor, and the family approaches you with what happened. They add that the patient also heard the comments. What would you do?

Name: _____ Date: _____

CHAPTER **10**

The Respiratory System

ADDITIONAL QUESTIONS

Multiple-Choice

Circle the best answer for each of the following questions.

1. Which of the following is not a part of the upper respiratory tract?

   a. nares

   b. turbinates

   c. pharynx

   d. alveoli

2. The medical term for windpipe is:

   a. trachea

   b. thyroid cartilage

   c. Adam's apple

   d. carini

3. The purpose of pleural fluid is to:

   a. reduce friction as an individual breathes

   b. moisten air passage

   c. filter debris

   d. reduce surface tension within the bronchioles

4. Which of the following statements is true about inspiration?

   a. For inspiration to take place, pressure in the thoracic cavity needs to decrease.

   b. For inspiration to take place, atmospheric pressure needs to be lower than thoracic pressure.

   c. For inspiration to take place, pressure in the thoracic cavity needs to increase.

   d. For inspiration to take place, atmospheric pressure and thoracic pressure need to be equal.

5. Which of the three sections of the pharynx conducts air, food, and liquid?

    a. oropharynx

    b. nasopharynx

    c. tracheopharynx

    d. all of the above

6. Directly below the Adam's apple is a large cartilage called the:

    a. thyroid cartilage

    b. epiglottis cartilage

    c. arytenoid cartilage

    d. cricoid cartilage

7. How does the epiglottis work during swallowing?

    a. As we breathe in, the epiglottis moves from its natural closed position to an open position so air can enter the larynx and trachea.

    b. As we swallow, the epiglottis flaps down to close off the larynx so food does not slip into that area.

    c. As we breathe in, the epiglottis closes off our esophagus so air does not enter into that area.

    d. It acts as a "guard gate," closing off the Eustachian tubes so air and food cannot enter and cause problems.

8. The function of the turbinates are to:

    a. warm and moisten air

    b. filter large particles

    c. trap oxygen so it remains in the airways

    d. prevent the entrance of carbon dioxide into the airways

9. The process of gas exchange in which carbon dioxide is removed from the blood and oxygen is added is called:

    a. internal respiration

    b. internal ventilation

    c. external respiration

    d. external ventilation

10. The bulk movement of air down to the lungs is termed:

    a. ventilation

    b. respiration

    c. transgasideous migration

    d. pulmonary peristalsis

11. Which of the following is not a function of the upper airway?

    a. heating and cooling of inspired air

    b. phonation

    c. olfaction

    d. external respiration

Matching 1

Match the following terms with their definitions.

_____	1. bronchioles	a.	lymphatic tissues found in the nasopharynx
_____	2. bronchi	b.	marks the end of the upper respiratory tract
_____	3. epiglottis	c.	bifurcation forming left and right mainstem bronchus
_____	4. erythropoiesis	d.	left lung region that corresponds to right middle lobe
_____	5. hemoglobin	e.	process of creating more blood cells
_____	6. vocal cords	f.	blood molecule that transports oxygen
_____	7. carini	g.	smaller airways
_____	8. lingula	h.	prevents food and liquid from entering the airway
_____	9. adenoids	i.	lightens the head
_____	10. sinuses	j.	larger airways

Matching 2

Match the following terms with their definitions.

_____	1. pleural effusion	a.	inflamed airways and large amounts of sputum
_____	2. tuberculosis	b.	constriction of the airway in response to an allergy
_____	3. emphysema	c.	fluid accumulation in the pleural space
_____	4. empyema	d.	infectious disease; vast lung damage can occur
_____	5. bronchospasm	e.	pus located in the pleural space
_____	6. asthma	f.	blood in the pleural space
_____	7. pneumothorax	g.	when the air sacs of the lungs are partially or totally collapsed
_____	8. atelectasis	h.	air in the thoracic cavity
_____	9. chronic bronchitis	i.	constriction of airways
_____	10. hemothorax	j.	irreversible condition in which air sacs become destroyed

Short Answer and Fill-in-the-Blank

1. How long will the oxygen reserve in your body normally last? _____

2. Approximately how many lungs full of air will you breathe in your lifetime? _____

3. When considering inhalation and exhalation, which is usually passive? _____

4. What is a patient who develops atelectasis *not* doing?

   _____

   _____

   _____

5. List the types of organisms that can cause pneumonia.

   _____

   _____

   _____

Labeling 1

Label the parts of the structures of the upper airway in the following figure.

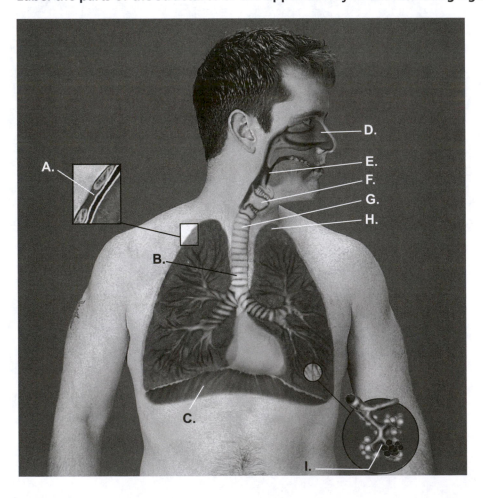

A. _____

B. _____

C. _____

D. _____

E. _____

F. _____

G. _____

H. _____

I. _____

Labeling 2

Label the structures of the respiratory system in the following figure.

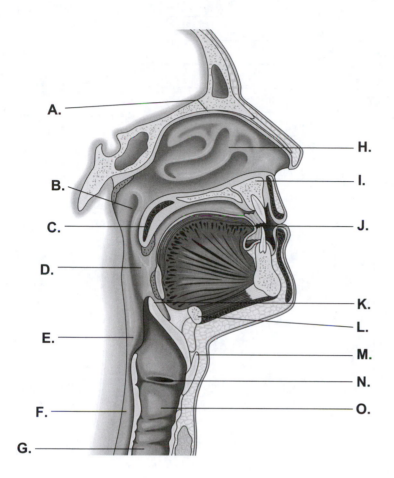

A. _____

B. _____

C. _____

D. _____

E. _____

F. _____

G. _____

H. _____

I. _____

J. _____

K. _____

L. _____

M. _____

N. _____

O. _____

Labeling 3

Label structures of the tracheobronchial tree in the following figure.

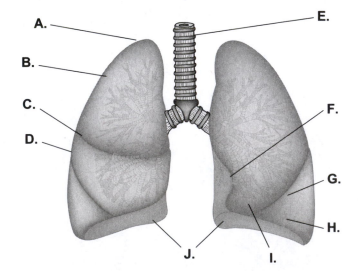

A. _____

B. _____

C. _____

D. _____

E. _____

F. _____

G. _____

H. _____

I. _____

Labeling 4

Label the structures and regions of the lungs in the following figure.

A. _____

B. _____

C. _____

D. _____

E. _____

F. _____

G. _____

H. _____

I. _____

J. _____

ADDITIONAL ACTIVITIES/LABS

1. Use your library or contact the American Lung Association to research the causes of lung disease. Create a poster for a school display explaining how to avoid respiratory problems or diseases.

2. After your teacher has paired the members of your class off, take turns assessing respiratory rates with your partner for a full minute. You will need either a watch with a sweep hand or a digital watch with a second display. The rate can be assessed by either observing the rise of the chest or by actually placing a hand on the chest. Note the ease or difficulty of concurrently monitoring the respiratory rate and the passage of time. Were you more conscious of your breathing as your partner monitored your respiratory rate? Could this affect your normal breathing pattern? Repeat the process, but this time change your breathing pattern or rate and see whether your partner notices the difference.

Extended Concepts

Central and Peripheral Chemoreceptors

How does your body know to speed your breathing when you play basketball or are running? Why don't you pant while sitting at your desk in school? Your peripheral and central chemoreceptors are the main influences on your ventilator patterns.

The most powerful stimulus for breathing is the concentration of hydrogen ions (H^+) in the cerebrospinal fluid (CSF). As the amount of carbon dioxide (CO_2) builds up in your blood, a chemical reaction causes the H^+ concentration to increase and move into the CSF. This alerts the central chemoreceptor in the brain to signal the respiratory component of the medulla to increase ventilation. As you breathe more rapidly and deeply, the CO_2 level in your body decreases. As the H^+ concentration decreases, the central receptors signal ventilation to slow down.

Peripheral receptors (also known as carotid and aortic bodies, due to their location) are oxygen-sensitive cells that influence ventilator patterns by monitoring the level of oxygen in the blood. As the oxygen level in the arteries (PaO_2) decreases, these receptors send a signal to the medulla to increase ventilation.

What Do You Think?

A growing body of evidence shows that a parent who smokes cigarettes in the home may increase a child's risk of developing respiratory diseases such as bronchitis and may increase the incidence of asthmatic attacks in an asthmatic child. Knowing this, if a parent continues smoking in an area of the home shared by a child and that child develops bronchitis, should the parent be arrested for child endangerment?

Name: _____   Date: _____

CHAPTER **11**

The Cardiovascular and Lymphatic Systems

ADDITIONAL QUESTIONS

Multiple-Choice

Circle the best answer for each of the following questions.

1. The valve between the right atria and right ventricles is the:

    a. bicuspid valve

    b. tricuspid valve

    c. pulmonary valve

    d. atrial valve

2. The blood cells that are responsible for protecting us against pathogens are:

    a. leukocytes

    b. thrombocytes

    c. platelets

    d. erythrocytes

3. Where in the chest is the heart located?

    a. directly in the middle of the chest, with apex above the base

    b. slightly right of center with the base resting on the diaphragm

    c. half to the right and half to the left of chest midline, with the base directly resting on the diaphragm

    d. slightly left of center with the base above the apex

4. The right side of the heart is responsible for:

    a. collecting and distributing oxygenated and deoxygenated blood to the right side of the body

    b. collecting deoxygenated blood from all over the body and sending it just to the lungs

    c. sending oxygenated blood to the upper body and collecting deoxygenated blood from the lower body

    d. sending deoxygenated blood to and collecting oxygenated blood from the lungs

5. The left side of the heart is responsible for:

   a. collecting and distributing deoxygenated blood to the left side of the body

   b. sending oxygenated blood to the lower body and collecting deoxygenated blood from the upper body

   c. collecting oxygenated blood from the lungs and sending it to the entire body

   d. sending deoxygenated blood to the lungs and collecting similar blood from the head

6. What prevents blood from rushing into the left atrium upon ventricular contraction?

   a. the third chamber, called the atrioventricular chamber

   b. a valve called the tricuspid

   c. a valve called the mitral

   d. decompression of the diaphragm

7. As fluid volume increases, what happens to blood pressure?

   a. it rises

   b. it falls

   c. it stays the same

   d. nothing, as there is no relationship between fluid volume and BP

8. Which of the following statements is true?

   a. The right ventricle sends blood to both the right and left lungs to pick up a fresh supply of oxygen.

   b. The left ventricle sends blood to both the right and left lungs to pick up a fresh supply of oxygen.

   c. The right ventricle sends blood to the right lung, and the left ventricle sends blood to the left lung to pick up a fresh supply of oxygen.

   d. The right and left atria direct blood to the right and left lungs respectively.

9. Correctly arrange the electrical pathway of the heart from where the impulse is initially generated to where it is carried to the contractile muscle cells.

   a. bundle of HIS, vagus nerve, sinoatrial node, atrioventricular node

   b. sinoatrial node, vagus nerve, Purkinje cells, atrioventricular node, bundle of HIS

   c. sinoatrial node, atrioventricular node, bundle of HIS, Purkinje fibers

   d. vagus nerve, sinoatrial node, atrioventricular node, Purkinje fibers, bundle of HIS

10. On the ECG, which of the waves represents the depolarization of the atria?

    a. T

    b. QRS

    c. It is masked by another wave

    d. P

11. The function of the spleen is to:

    a. produce red blood cells before birth

    b. filter pathogens from the bloodstream

    c. remove iron from hemoglobin

    d. all the above

12. Lymphatic trunks empty into:

    a. collecting ducts

    b. subclavian veins

    c. lymph nodes

    d. thymus

13. Where is the spleen located?

    a. between the heart and the sternum

    b. upper right quadrant of abdomen

    c. upper left quadrant of pelvis

    d. upper left quadrant of abdomen

Matching 1

Match the following terms with their definitions.

_____ 1. veins

_____ 2. phagocytosis

_____ 3. erythrocytes

_____ 4. arteries

_____ 5. leukocytes

_____ 6. neutrophils

_____ 7. thrombocytes

_____ 8. eosinophils

a. moves blood away from heart

b. WBCs functioning to combat parasites and decrease allergies

c. the process by which a cell surrounds and ingests an invader

d. collective term for white blood cells

e. collective term for red blood cells

f. cells that perform phagocytosis

g. platelets

h. moves blood toward heart

Matching 2

Match the following terms with their definitions.

_____ 1. angina pectoris

_____ 2. ischemia

_____ 3. heart failure

_____ 4. endocarditis

_____ 5. prolapse

_____ 6. myocardial infarction

_____ 7. atherosclerosis

_____ 8. arteriosclerosis

a. the ventricles are not pumping blood efficiently

b. accumulation of plaque in vessels

c. radiating chest pain due to decreased cardiac blood flow

d. heart tissue injury due to low oxygen levels

e. hardening of the blood vessels

f. failure of heart valve closure

g. heart attack

h. inflammation of the lining of the heart

Short Answer and Fill-in-the-Blank

1. The _____ is a smooth layer of tissue that also forms the valves of the heart.

2. All of the blood that circulates in the body will eventually return to the heart through the _____ _____ _____ or the _____ _____ _____.

3. The main pacemaker of the heart is known as the _____ _____.

4. Why is the blood in the pulmonary artery not the same as blood in the other arteries?

_____

_____

_____

5. Which side of the heart pumps blood to the body? _____

6. _____ is a term used to describe an inflammation of the heart muscle.

7. What condition results from reduced blood flow to the heart tissue and causes pain or a heavy sensation in the chest that can radiate to the shoulder or arm? _____ _____

8. The condition wherein a heart valve attempts to close but falls backward and allows blood to "squirt" backward is known as a _____.

9. _____ is the fluid portion of blood.

Labeling 1

Label the structures of the heart in the following figure.

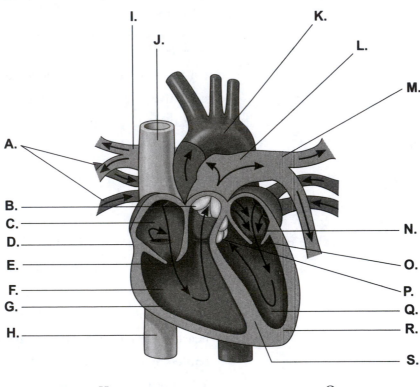

A. _____	H. _____	O. _____
B. _____	I. _____	P. _____
C. _____	J. _____	Q. _____
D. _____	K. _____	R. _____
E. _____	L. _____	S. _____
F. _____	M. _____	
G. _____	N. _____	

Labeling 2

Label the conduction system of the heart in the following figure.

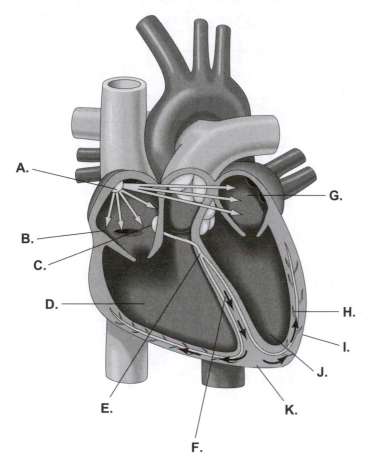

A. _____

B. _____

C. _____

D. _____

E. _____

F. _____

G. _____

H. _____

I. _____

J. _____

K. _____

Labeling 3

Label the vessels and organs of the lymphatic system in the following figure.

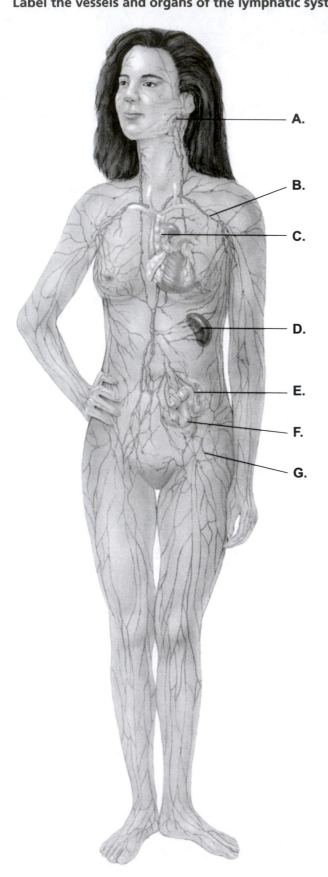

A. _____

B. _____

C. _____

D. _____

E. _____

F. _____

G. _____

A.

B.

C.

D.

E.

F.

G.

Labeling 4

Label the principal lymphatic trunks of the body in the following figure.

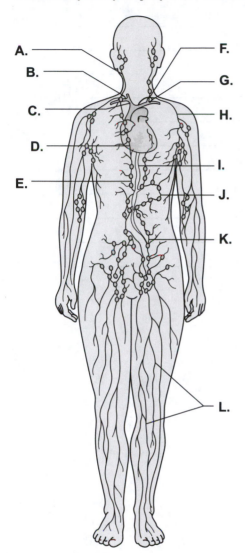

A. _____

B. _____

C. _____

D. _____

E. _____

F. _____

G. _____

H. _____

I. _____

J. _____

K. _____

L. _____

Labeling 5

Label the following figure showing the relationship between the cardiovascular and lymphatic systems.

A. _____

B. _____

C. _____

D. _____

E. _____

F. _____

G. _____

H. _____

I. _____

J. _____

K. _____

ADDITIONAL ACTIVITIES/LABS

1. After obtaining a cow's heart from a butcher shop, take turns dissecting and labeling the various parts of the heart.

2. After your teacher divides the class into groups, research lifestyles that promote a healthy heart. Design and create posters for your school to educate students regarding these lifestyles.

Extended Concepts

At some time during your school career, you have probably heard the term *mononucleosis*, but what exactly is it? Mononucleosis is an infectious disease characterized by an increased number of mononuclear leukocytes (white blood cells possessing only one nucleus each) in the blood and tissues.

This disease causes swollen lymph glands, sore throat, malaise, skin rash, and fever, and is caused by the Epstein-Barr virus. Sometimes there is liver inflammation which can lead to jaundice (a yellowing of the skin). Victims are usually young adults aged 15 to 30, but cases can occur in children.

Mononucleosis is sometimes called the "kissing disease" because the virus is found in the victim's saliva and can thus be spread via oral contact.

The severity of the disease ranges from mild to severe, with death rarely occurring. Although bed rest is often suggested for those suffering from mononucleosis, no specific treatment has yet been discovered.

What Do You Think?

Certain religions will not allow natural blood transfusions under any circumstances. A severely ill patient who possesses such religious beliefs requires a transfusion to live. Are there any alternatives to save the patient while not violating the patient's beliefs? How would you handle this situation?

CHAPTER **12**

The Gastrointestinal System

ADDITIONAL QUESTIONS

Multiple-Choice

Circle the best answer for each of the following questions.

1. Which of the following is NOT a major GI structure?

   a. stomach

   b. esophagus

   c. oral cavity

   d. spleen

2. These substances speed up the chemical process of breaking down food.

   a. enzymes

   b. proteins

   c. glucose

   d. fructose

3. Arrange the segments of the large intestine in the order waste travels through:

   a. cecum, descending colon, ascending colon, transverse colon, sigmoid colon, rectum

   b. cecum, ascending colon, transverse colon, descending colon, sigmoid colon, rectum

   c. sigmoid colon, ascending colon, transverse colon, descending colon, cecum, rectum

   d. sigmoid colon, descending colon, ascending colon, transverse colon, cecum, rectum

4. Where does the majority of absorption of usable nutrients take place?

   a. stomach

   b. mouth

   c. large intestine

   d. small intestine

5. Which sphincter lies between the stomach and small intestine?

   a. cardiac

   b. gastroenteral

   c. pyloric

   d. ileocecal

6. What is the function of the liver?

   a. detoxify blood

   b. produce clotting factors

   c. maintain proper glucose levels

   d. all of the above

7. What is a *lacteal,* and where is it located?

   a. lymphatic capillary in each villus of small intestine

   b. blood capillary beside goblet cells in the pancreas

   c. enzyme in the pancreas that, when secreted, digests milk

   d. mucous lining found in the stomach

8. Using the cardiac sphincter as a reference point, where is the fundus of the stomach?

   a. left, superior

   b. right, inferior

   c. left, inferior

   d. right, superior

9. The uvula is associated with which structure?

   a. soft palate

   b. hard palate

   c. tongue

   d. pharynx

10. What substance starts chemically breaking down in the mouth due to salivary secretions?

    a. starch

    b. protein

    c. fat

    d. lactose

Matching 1

Match the following terms with their definitions.

_____ 1. cirrhosis

_____ 2. peptic ulcer

_____ 3. peritonitis

_____ 4. cholelithiasis

_____ 5. hepatitis B

_____ 6. heartburn

_____ 7. gingivitis

_____ 8. gastritis

_____ 9. ascites

_____ 10. cholecystitis

a. general term for an abnormal amount of fluid in the peritoneal cavity

b. inflammation of the stomach

c. chronic disease of the liver

d. inflammation of the gallbladder

e. backup of gastric juices into esophagus

f. gall stones

g. often located in stomach/duodenum, caused by pathogens and stress

h. inflammation of serous membrane lining abdominal cavity

i. inflammation of the gums

j. potential life-threatening viral disease

Matching 2

Match the following terms with their definitions.

_____ 1. esophagus

_____ 2. stomach

_____ 3. small intestine

_____ 4. large intestine

_____ 5. oral cavity

_____ 6. gallbladder

_____ 7. liver

_____ 8. pancreas

_____ 9. salivary gland

_____ 10. appendix

a. unknown function

b. most digestion and absorption

c. releases digestive enzymes into duodenum

d. begins starch digestion and mechanical breakdown of food

e. secretes enzyme that digests starch

f. stores bile

g. makes bile

h. makes and stores feces

i. transports food to stomach, no digestion

j. stores food, digests protein

Short Answer and Fill-in-the-Blank

1. The _____ _____ is the name given to the 30-foot tube through which food travels in the body.

2. The accessory organs are the _____, _____, and _____.

3. Digestion requires both _____ and _____ activity.

4. Another term for fats is _____.

5. What is the function of the papilla, located on the tongue?

_____

_____

_____

6. What is the function of incisors?

_____

_____

_____

7. The _____ is a small, narrow tube approximately 3 inches long and attached to the large intestine.

8. What is the importance of vitamin K?

_____

_____

_____

9. When considering carbohydrates and fats, which are digested more rapidly and why?

_____

_____

_____

Labeling 1

Label the organs and structures of the gastrointestinal system in the following figure. Include any applicable combining forms.

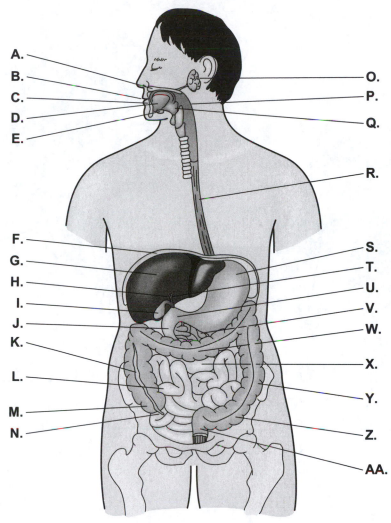

A. _____	J. _____	S. _____
B. _____	K. _____	T. _____
C. _____	L. _____	U. _____
D. _____	M. _____	V. _____
E. _____	N. _____	W. _____
F. _____	O. _____	X. _____
G. _____	P. _____	Y. _____
H. _____	Q. _____	Z. _____
I. _____	R. _____	AA. _____

Labeling 2

Label the structures of the stomach in the following figure.

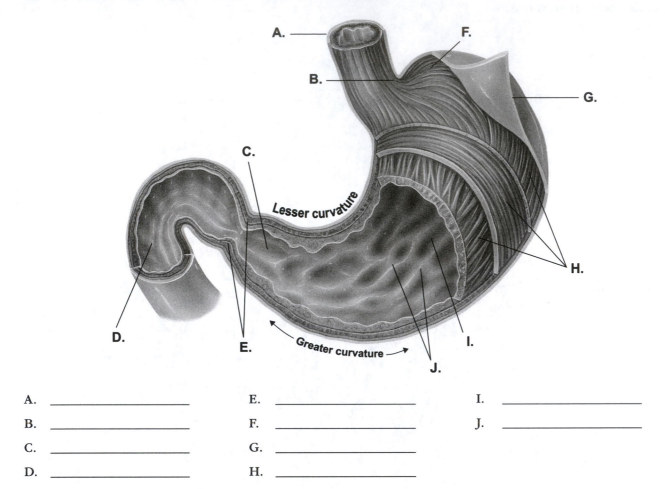

A. _____   E. _____   I. _____

B. _____   F. _____   J. _____

C. _____   G. _____

D. _____   H. _____

Labeling 3

Label the large intestine in the following figure.

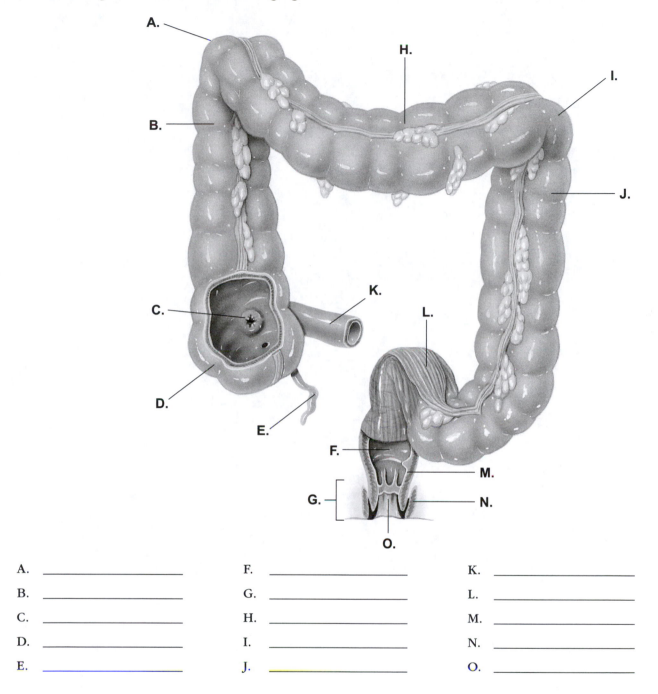

A. _____	F. _____	K. _____
B. _____	G. _____	L. _____
C. _____	H. _____	M. _____
D. _____	I. _____	N. _____
E. _____	J. _____	O. _____

ADDITIONAL ACTIVITIES/LABS

1. Keep a record of what you eat during one week. The next week, examine this record to determine whether you are fulfilling the daily requirements for the various food groups. If you are not, create a proper diet for the next week. How hard or easy was it to follow your new diet? Discuss your findings in class.

2. Make a list of foods you consider to be high in protein, fat, or carbohydrates. Then go shopping, review the labels of these foods, and determine the accuracy of your predictions.

Extended Concepts

We have all had stomach problems at one time or another. *Gastritis* is the term used to describe inflammation of the stomach lining. Symptoms of gastritis can include discomfort after eating, loss of appetite, nausea, and vomiting.

Gastritis can be traced to a number of causes including infections caused by either viruses or bacteria, drugs, alcohol, corrosive substances, or allergies. Chronic gastritis can result from ulcers or iron-deficiency anemia.

What Do You Think?

You have likely heard or read about eating disorders such as anorexia nervosa and bulimia. Why do you think such disorders are on the rise in modern society? What do you think can be done to reverse this trend?

CHAPTER **13**

The Urinary and Reproductive Systems

ADDITIONAL QUESTIONS

Multiple-Choice

Circle the best answer for each of the following questions.

1. Which of the following is NOT a major structure of the urinary system?

    a. kidneys

    b. testes

    c. ureters

    d. urethra

2. The urinary bladder walls are composed of what type of muscle?

    a. involuntary

    b. voluntary

    c. skeletal

    d. b and c

3. Which of the urinary organs transports urine from the kidneys to the bladder?

    a. nephrons

    b. urethra

    c. ureters

    d. glomerulus

4. In which layer of the kidney is blood filtered?

    a. pelvis

    b. medulla

    c. cortex

    d. capsule

5. Approximately how many nephrons are in each kidney?

   a. 2

   b. 100,000

   c. 10,000

   d. 1,000,000

6. BPH is a pathology marked by:

   a. breast polyps commonly seen in women over 50

   b. biological pelvic heliobacterium that affects pre-puberty girls

   c. prostate enlargement commonly seen in males over 50

   d. hermaphroditic pelvic organs caused by fetal hormone imbalance

7. The primary male reproductive organ is/are the:

   a. testes

   b. ureters

   c. sperm

   d. muscles

8. At what point is the developing human referred to as a fetus?

   a. at fertilization

   b. 4 weeks after fertilization until birth

   c. at implantation

   d. 12 weeks after fertilization until birth

9. Which highly sensitive structure of the female anatomy has great similarity to the penis and becomes erectile during sexual arousal?

   a. breast

   b. ovaries

   c. mons pubis

   d. clitoris

10. Which hormones are produced by the ovaries?

    a. estrogen

    b. testosterone

    c. progesterone

    d. a and c

Matching 1

Match the following terms with their definitions.

____ 1. fallopian tube   a. where fetus develops

____ 2. vagina   b. secretes estrogen and progesterone

____ 3. ovary   c. birth canal

____ 4. uterus   d. where fertilization takes place

____ 5. scrotum   e. houses the testes

____ 6. bulbourethral glands   f. where sperm develop

____ 7. testes   g. thick mucous secretion that acts like a lubricant

Matching 2

Match the following terms with their definitions.

____ 1. ureter   a. bean-shaped structure that filters blood and forms urine

____ 2. urethra   b. functional unit of the kidney

____ 3. kidney   c. contains water, wastes, glucose, and electrolytes

____ 4. bladder   d. transports urine from kidneys to bladder

____ 5. nephron   e. transports urine to outside the body

____ 6. Bowman's capsule   f. nitrogenous waste

____ 7. filtrate   g. where filtration of blood occurs

____ 8. urea   h. hollow holding structure for urine

Short Answer and Fill-in-the-Blank

1. List the main structures of the urinary system: _____, _____, _____, _____.

2. Filtration by the kidneys is accomplished by microscopic structures called _____.

3. Urine is approximately 95% _____.

4. List the male reproductive organs: _____, _____, _____.

5. List the female reproductive organs: _____, _____, _____, _____.

6. Fertilization actually occurs in the _____ _____.

7. The uterus is also known as the _____.

8. Another name for kidney stones is _____.

9. Prostate cancer is a common cancer in _____ who are _____ years of age or older.

Labeling 1

Label the organs of the urinary system in the following figure.

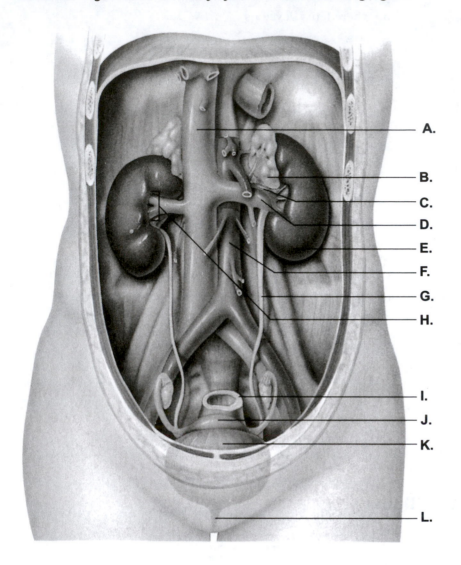

A. _____

B. _____

C. _____

D. _____

E. _____

F. _____

G. _____

H. _____

I. _____

J. _____

K. _____

L. _____

Labeling 2

Label the organs and structures of the male reproductive system in the following figure.

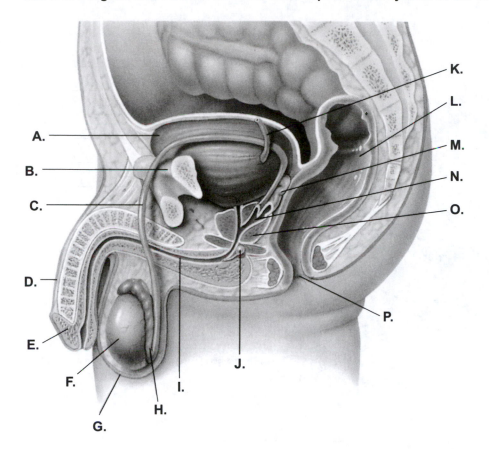

A. _____

B. _____

C. _____

D. _____

E. _____

F. _____

G. _____

H. _____

I. _____

J. _____

K. _____

L. _____

M. _____

N. _____

O. _____

P. _____

Labeling 3

Label the organs and structures of the female reproductive system in the following figure. Include any applicable combining forms.

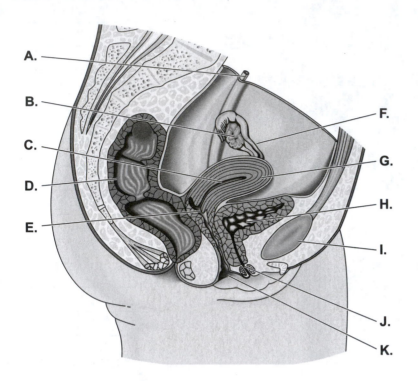

A. _____

B. _____

C. _____

D. _____

E. _____

F. _____

G. _____

H. _____

I. _____

J. _____

K. _____

L. _____

M. _____

N. _____

O. _____

P. _____

Q. _____

R. _____

S. _____

T. _____

U. _____

V. _____

Genitalia

ADDITIONAL ACTIVITIES/LABS

1. Construct a model kidney out of everyday materials such as PVC tubing and yarn, cardboard tubing, or filters; be creative. Label and demonstrate the functions of the system parts.

2. Research the importance of prenatal care and write a report or make a poster illustrating your findings.

Extended Concepts

The *glucose tolerance test* is used to determine whether an individual has diabetes mellitus (abnormal metabolism of glucose). Generally, the testing procedure requires that the patient eat nothing for 18 to 24 hours prior to the test. The patient then drinks a concentrated solution of glucose. Levels of glucose in both the blood and urine are measured at certain time intervals (usually ½, 1, 2, and 3 hours) after the solution is ingested.

The glucose concentration of a healthy individual will rise to almost twice the normal level within the first hour. The level will then return to normal within 2 hours. Very little, if any, glucose will be excreted in the patient's urine. An individual with diabetes mellitus, however, will display a much greater rise in glucose concentration level, the return to a normal level will take longer (three or more hours), and a large amount of glucose will be excreted in the patient's urine. As you already know, this response to the glucose tolerance test is caused by the diabetic's lack of the hormone insulin, which is needed for the removal of glucose.

What Do You Think?

Genetic engineering has been used for years to produce healthier and hardier plants. In animal husbandry, genetic manipulation has increased yields of meat and milk. Genetic engineering has also directly benefited humans. For example, humulin, a genetically designed form of human insulin, has made life much easier for many thousands of patients suffering from diabetes. What do you think about genetic engineering? What are the potential hazards or abuses?

Fundamentals of Mathematics

C H A P T E R **14**

Basic Mathematical Definitions and Fractions

ADDITIONAL QUESTIONS

1. Rewrite each of the following fractions in lowest terms.

   a. $\frac{24}{32} =$ _____

   b. $\frac{3}{15} =$ _____

   c. $\frac{15}{25} =$ _____

   d. $\frac{0}{4} =$ _____

2. Rewrite each of the following fractions as a higher equivalent fraction.

   a. $\frac{2}{3} = \frac{}{21}$

   b. $\frac{1}{2} = \frac{}{210}$

   c. $\frac{4}{5} = \frac{}{35}$

   d. $\frac{5}{8} = \frac{}{64}$

3. Rewrite each of the following as a whole or mixed number; simplify as necessary.

   a. $\frac{12}{3} =$ _____

   b. $\frac{15}{2} =$ _____

   c. $\frac{24}{10} =$ _____

   d. $\frac{39}{12} =$ _____

4. Rewrite each of the following as an improper fraction.

   a. $6\frac{1}{3} =$ _____

   b. $2\frac{4}{5} =$ _____

   c. $3\frac{4}{7} =$ _____

   d. $4\frac{7}{8} =$ _____

5. Add or subtract and simplify each of the following.

   a. $\frac{1}{5} + \frac{3}{5} =$ _____

   b. $\frac{7}{15} + \frac{8}{15} =$ _____

   c. $\frac{9}{10} - \frac{3}{10} =$ _____

   d. $\frac{2}{3} + \frac{1}{5} =$ _____

   e. $\frac{3}{7} - \frac{1}{4} =$ _____

   f. $\frac{9}{16} - \frac{1}{2} =$ _____

6. Multiply and simplify each of the following.

   a. $\dfrac{3}{4} \times \dfrac{2}{3} =$ _____

   b. $\dfrac{1}{4} \times \dfrac{2}{5} =$ _____

   c. $\dfrac{5}{6} \times \dfrac{16}{25} =$ _____

   d. $\dfrac{3}{14} \times \dfrac{7}{9} =$ _____

7. Find the reciprocals for each of the following.

   a. $\dfrac{2}{3} =$ _____

   b. $\dfrac{3}{4} =$ _____

   c. 2 _____

8. Divide and simplify each of the following.

   a. $\dfrac{2}{3} \div \dfrac{4}{9} =$ _____

   b. $5 \div \dfrac{10}{3} =$ _____

   c. $\dfrac{8}{5} \div 16 =$ _____

   d. $\dfrac{17}{28} \div \dfrac{51}{62} =$ _____

9. A health care professional was asked to administer 750 units of a medication. However, all that is in stock are bottles containing 125 units. How many bottles must be administered? Express the answer as a mixed number.

10. A patient is given 3/4 tablespoon of medication before lunch and 3/8 tablespoon after lunch. How much total medication did the patient receive?

11. Three bottles of the same medication have been opened. They are 1/4, 5/8 and 1/2 of their original amounts. If added together, will they fit into 2 bottles?

12. A bottle is half full. A health care provider is to give 2/3 of the remaining bottle. How much of the original bottle does this represent?

13. A bottle contains 800 tablets. A pharmacy technician is asked to supply three-fourths of them to the nurse's station. How many should be sent?

14. Suppose you have 3/8 of a bottle of medication left. If each dose is 1/16 of a bottle, to find the number of doses remaining in the bottle, find 3/8 ÷ 1/16.

ADDITIONAL ACTIVITIES/LABS

1. Bring in articles from the newspaper or magazines that use fractions, and discuss why it is important to use fractions. That is, why use fractions in those instances, instead of other types of numbers?

2. Attempt to determine the rules for divisibility by the numbers 2, 10, 5, and 3. For example, all numbers that are divisible by 2 end in _____, _____, _____, _____ or _____.

Extended Concepts

Reynolds Number

If you turn on a faucet so that the water comes out of it in a steady stream, you will observe what is called *laminar flow*. As you turn the faucet so that the water flow increases, you will notice that the water begins to break apart at the end of the steady stream. This is known as *turbulent flow*. If you look at the smoke rising from a cigarette, you will notice both of these occurrences. At first, the flow of smoke will be steady (laminar flow), and then the flow will change to a less stable flow (turbulent flow) and little circular currents, called *eddies*, will begin to form.

Whether the flow through a tube, such as a bronchial tube, is laminar or turbulent depends on several factors. They are:

> p, the fluid density
> v, the speed at which the gas or liquid is moving
> D, the diameter of the tube
> n, the viscosity (thickness) of the gas or liquid

The Reynolds number is a fractional quantity that can be used to describe whether flow will be laminar or turbulent. A Reynolds number of 2,000 or less means the flow will be laminar; a Reynolds number of more than 4,000 means the flow will be turbulent. For values between 2,000 and 4,000, the flow has some qualities of both and is considered to be *turbulaminar.*

The formula for determining the Reynolds number (R), using the letters, is:

$$R = \frac{pvD}{n}$$

Some Reynolds's numbers for your airways might be as follows:

> mouth: 2,986
> trachea: 3,513
> primary bronchi: 2,930
> bronchiole: 47
> terminal bronchiole: 3

What Do You Think?

You are the chief executive officer of an urban hospital. One of your many responsibilities is to go out and obtain financial contributors. One such contributor has offered $6 million for the establishment of a breast cancer clinic. There are four other breast cancer clinics in the city. When you alert the potential contributor to this fact, she says, "Well, we'll just have to make ours the best, and we'll blow the competition out of the water!" During this same period of time, you discover that the city lacks other programs and services, including a prenatal clinic for prospective mothers, classes on parenting, and a controversial program of needle exchanges for IV drug users. You now have a choice: Do you take the $6 million for the breast cancer clinic, or do you ask the potential contributor to designate the money for these other identified needs? How can controversial programs impact financial contributions? How would you present your request to this potential contributor?

CHAPTER **15**

Decimals, Percents, and Ratios

ADDITIONAL QUESTIONS

1. Estimate the answer for each of the following, and then use a calculator to obtain a more precise answer.

	ESTIMATE	EXACT
a. $\dfrac{16.35}{5} =$	_____	_____
b. $7.23 + 6.1 + 9.355$	_____	_____
c. 2.03×6.55	_____	_____
d. $163.5 \div 7.05$	_____	_____

2. Complete the following table.

	FRACTION	DECIMAL	PERCENT
a.	$\frac{1}{5}$	_____	_____
b.	_____	_____	$16\frac{2}{3}\%$
c.	$\frac{3}{8}$	_____	_____
d.	_____	0 .75	_____
e.	_____	_____	35%
f.	_____	0 .125	_____

3. Thimerosal, in concentrations ranging from 0.0025% to 0.1%, is used for wet dressings. Express each as a common fraction, and as a decimal numeral.

_____

_____

4. Each nurse in a department receives an annual salary of $34,235.15. What is the total salary cost for this department if there are 12 nurses in the department?

_____

5. A hospital borrowed $3,325,050.36 to buy a new machine. If this loan is to be paid back in 3 years, with no interest, what is the monthly payment?

_____

6. A medical procedure costs $324.51 for 3 hours. How much does the procedure cost per hour?
_____ per minute?_____

7. Each pill given to a patient costs $1.35. If the patient is to be hospitalized for five days, and must take one pill three times a day while hospitalized, what will be the total cost of this medication? _____

8. What is 20% of 140?

_____

_____

9. What is 30% of 150?

_____

_____

10. What is 40% of 200?

_____

_____

11. A full bottle of liquid medicine has 800 units. If a doctor orders that 25% be administered, how many units were used? How much remains?

_____

_____

12. There are 1,600 tablets in a bottle. A pharmacist wants 20% of them to be packaged into smaller containers. How many must be repackaged? If there are 50 in each smaller package, how many of such packages will there be?

_____

_____

13. A physician ordered 160 syringes for his office. However, when they were delivered, she found that $37\frac{1}{2}$% were broken. How many syringes were usable?

_____

_____

14. A scientific study considers people who are 20% above their ideal body weight to be overweight. If you weigh 200 pounds and have an ideal body weight of 175 pounds, are you considered overweight according to this study?

_____

_____

15. If 24 cans of a beverage cost $8.00, while 30 cans cost $9.00, which is the better buy?

_____

_____

ADDITIONAL ACTIVITIES/LABS

1. List all the ways that decimals and percentages are used in baseball; for example, fielding percentage and earned-run average.

2. Cut pieces of string to different lengths. Use the pieces of string to form circles of different diameters. Measure the length of each string, and the diameter of the circle formed by the string. The ratio of the circle (i.e., the length of string) to the diameter should be approximately 3.14, because $\pi = \frac{c}{d}$.

Extended Concepts

Estimating Percentage of Burn

Care of and survival predictions for burn patients depend primarily on three variables:

- percent of body surface burned

- degree of the burn

- patient's vital signs

Although there are many ways to determine the percent of body surface burned, perhaps the most basic way is to use the "rule of nine" (see the figure below). According to the rule of nine, the entire head is 9% of the body surface area; each arm is 9%; each leg is twice 9%, or 18%; the chest and stomach together are 18%; the back is 18%; and the pelvic region is 1%.

So, for example, if a patient had burns over the entire back (18%), the back of the left arm (1/2 of 9%, or 4.5%), and the back of the left leg (1/2 of 18%, or 9%), a quick estimate of the body surface burned would be 18% + 4.5% + 9%, or 31.5%, which is roughly one-third (33%) of the patient's body surface.

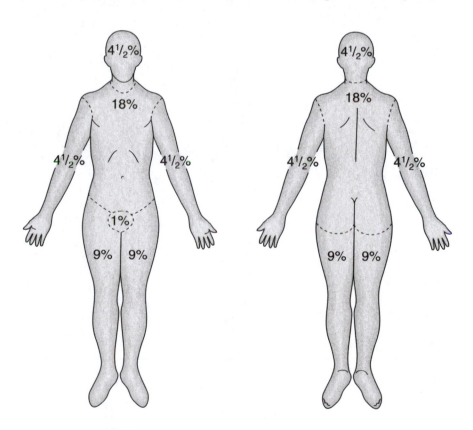

What Do You Think?

You work at a state mental institution that receives a large sum of money from the federal government to keep the institution operating. Several patients in your care have been selected for testing of a drug that is reported to intensify the body's ability to combat viral infections. If this drug works per the manufacturer claims, millions of lives might be saved worldwide. Side effects of the drug on humans are unknown. Oddly, the patients that were selected are all mentally incompetent and have no relatives. You ask your superior whether release or consent forms have been completed for these patients. Your superior states that "everything has been taken care of." What would you do next? Are any ethical issues inherent in this case? How do you weigh such things as "the good of the many," "informed consent," and "the ends justify the means?" Do you know of any similar real-life situations?

Name: _____ Date: _____

Exponents, Scientific Notation, and the Metric System

ADDITIONAL QUESTIONS

1. Evaluate each of the following.

   a. $2^4 =$ _____   b. $6^3 =$ _____   c. $10^5 =$ _____

2. Evaluate each of the following.

   a. $2^{-2} =$ _____   b. $3^{-4} =$ _____   c. $10^{-2} =$ _____

3. Write each of the following in scientific notation.

   a. $23{,}100{,}000 =$ _____   c. $0.000023 =$ _____

   b. $4{,}020{,}000{,}000 =$ _____   d. $0.0000104 =$ _____

4. Write each of the following in decimal form.

   a. $3 \times 10^6 =$ _____   c. $6.11 \times 10^{-9} =$ _____

   b. $4.02 \times 10^{-6} =$ _____   d. $732 \times 10^5 =$ _____

5. Light travels at a speed of 186,000 miles per second. How far does it travel in 1 minute? Write your answer in scientific notation. _____

6. The mass of an electron is 0.00000000000000000000000000911 grams. Write this number in scientific notation. _____

7. Convert each of the following to the units noted.

   a. $16\ \text{m} =$ _____ mm   c. $10{,}000\ \text{mg} =$ _____ g

   b. $6.33\ \text{kL} =$ _____ mL   d. $230{,}000\ \text{mL} =$ _____ L

8. Convert each of the following to the units noted.

   a. $2\ \text{days} =$ _____ min   c. $2\ \text{kg} =$ _____ cg

   b. $12.5\ \text{ft} =$ _____ in.   d. $12\ \text{lb} =$ _____ oz

9. Convert each of the following to the units noted.

    a. 200 g = _____ oz   c. 10 mi = _____ km

    b. 20 L = _____ qt   d. 2 in. = _____ cm

10. A medium-sized artery has a diameter of 3.4 mm. What does this equal in inches? _____

11. A human male's heart weighs approximately 340 g. What does this equal in pounds? _____

12. The capacity of the right atrium of the aorta is approximately 57 mL. What does this equal in ounces? _____

13. A white blood cell count is typically about 7,500,000,000/L blood. Express this in scientific notation.

    _____

    _____

14. The diameter of a proton is about 10^{-15} of a meter. Express this as a decimal.

    _____

    _____

15. An eosinophil is a type of white blood cell. If a patient's eosinophil count is 1.2×10^8 per liter, express it as a decimal.

    _____

    _____

16. How many mL are there in 2 quarts of hydrochloric acid?

    _____

    _____

17. How many mL are there in 6 quarts of saline?

    _____

    _____

18. How many ounces are there in 60 mL of solvent?

    _____

    _____

19. A blood sample has a glucose value of 75 mg/dL. Convert this to grams per liter.

    _____

    _____

20. Convert 20 miles per gallon to kilometers per gallon.

    _____

    _____

ADDITIONAL ACTIVITIES/LABS

1. After your teacher divides the class into groups, use mental math to find the answers to problems such as 3,000 × 500 and 10 × 52,000. Take turns with those in your group, and verbalize your thought processes. See whether you become better with practice.

2. The metric system is used in every large country except the United States. Estimate the metric measurements of various items in your home. Then, use a metric stick to measure those items. Compare your estimated and actual measurements.

3. Using an encyclopedia, research facts that are written, or could be written, in scientific notation. For example, the number of miles each planet is from the sun. Share your findings with the class.

Extended Concepts

Ideal Gases

Although a future chapter of the text is devoted entirely to gas laws, it might be appropriate to mention the *ideal gas law* now. A given quantity of gas does not have a definite volume, but rather expands to fill any container into which it is placed. There is, however, a direct relationship between the volume (V), temperature (T), pressure (P), and quantity (n) of a gas, expressed by the formula $PV = nRT$, and sometimes called the *general gas law*. This law describes the relationship between volume, temperature, pressure, and quantity for all gases. The value R is a constant, which is the same for all ideal gases. Rewritten, the formula becomes:

$$R = \frac{PV}{nT}$$

This constant is the same for all gases under ideal conditions. For example, suppose $P = 101{,}000$, $V = 0.0224$, $T = 273$, and $n = 1$. Then R becomes:

$$\frac{(101{,}000 \times 0.0224)}{(273 \times 1)}$$

or approximately 8.3. This is known as the *universal gas constant*. If the temperature of this given amount of gas, in this given space, were to rise to $T = 333$, the pressure would rise to 123,389 to compensate, and R would be: $\frac{(123{,}389 \times 0.224)}{(333 \times 1)}$, or approximately 8.3 again. This will be true for all gases.

What Do You Think?

You have been working closely with a physician who is well known and very well liked in the community. When you first met with this doctor several years ago, you were very impressed with her ability to relate to patients. Within a year, however, you noted occasional mistakes on her part, such as slightly inaccurate doses being prescribed for a given medication. These mistakes were always caught, and no patients were hurt. The doctor even joked about needing "to go back to high school" to improve her math skills.

During the past two years, however, there has been a drastic increase in the number and severity of these mistakes. Word is out that all of this doctor's patient orders should be double-checked by the hospital staff before being implemented. In addition, the doctor misdiagnosed a patient as having a simple recurring right-middle-lobe pneumonia. After 9 months of unsuccessful treatment, a specialist was brought in. The specialist immediately determined that the patient was suffering from a cancerous lung airway tumor that had spread throughout the body.

The doctor who is making these mistakes either chews gum or uses breath mints constantly. While talking with her one day, you could have sworn that you smelled a slight hint of alcohol. She considers you a trusted colleague and friend. What should you do?

CHAPTER **17**

An Introduction to Algebra

ADDITIONAL QUESTIONS

Short Answer and Fill-in-the-Blank

1. Simplify each of the following.

   a. $2 + 6 \times 3 =$ _____

   b. $(2 + 3)^2 - 7 \times 2 =$ _____

   c. $2 - (-3) + (-1) =$ _____

   d. $(-2)(-3) + 5 =$ _____

   e. $(2 + 3)^2/(2 - 7) - (3)^2 =$ _____

   f. $(-3)(5)-(-2)(-6)-(-1)(6) =$ _____

   g. $(2 - 4)^2 - (-12/-3)^2 =$ _____

2. Using the values given, evaluate each of the following.

   a. $3(p - q) + 2p$, if $p = 3$ and $q = -1$ _____

   b. $5/9(F - 32)$, if $F = 32$ _____

   c. $9/5C + 32$, if $C = 100$ _____

3. In each of the following, circle the terms (if any) that are similar to $3x$.

   a. $3xy - 2x + 7y$ c. $3y^2 + xy + x$

   b. $2x^2 - 3x + 7$ d. $x^2y^3 - 6xy + y$

4. Simplify each of the following.

   a. $6x - 3x + 2y + 1$ _____   c. $7(x - 1) + 2(3x - 2)$ _____

   b. $2(x + y) - 3x$ _____   d. $2(3y - 6) - 4(y + 1)$ _____

5. Write variable expressions for each of the following.

   a. x minus 7 _____

   b. y times 3 _____

   c. 2 more than p _____

   d. 10 less than x _____

   e. m divided by 2 _____

   f. the ratio of p and q _____

6. If *x* represents the number of pills taken from a bottle, what expression represents the number of pills remaining in the bottle, if a full bottle contains 50 pills? _____

7. A patient had a total fluid intake of 2,000 mL yesterday. According to her chart, she had output of 1,250 mL in the morning and 700 mL in the afternoon. Did she gain or lose fluid for the day?

_____

_____

8. A patient had a total fluid intake of 1,200 mL yesterday. According to her chart, she had output of 250, 750, and 225 mL today. Did she gain or lose fluid for the day?

_____

_____

9. A resident at an extended care facility had a total fluid intake of 1,800 mL yesterday. According to his chart, today he had outputs of 150 mL, 200 mL, 300 mL, 450 mL, and 350 mL. Did he gain or lose fluid for the day?

_____

_____

10. Pick a number. Add six. Triple the result. Subtract eighteen. Divide by three. Is the number the same as that with which you started? Do it again with a different number. Write an algebraic expression that describes why this happens.

_____

_____

ADDITIONAL ACTIVITIES/LABS

1. Using the numbers 1, 2, 3, and 4, in order, combine them using parentheses and the operations of addition, subtraction, multiplication, and division to obtain the largest possible value, for example, $(1 + 2) \times (3 + 4) = 21$. *Hint:* The real answer is 36.

2. Repeat activity number 1 to find the smallest possible value, which is 0.

3. Use a newspaper to select a stock on the New York Stock Exchange. After following its gains and losses for 5 days, predict whether the stock will gain or lose the next week.

Extended Concepts

Intravenous Delivery System

Intravenous (IV) administration delivers drugs via drops over an extended time period. The advantages of delivering a drug one drop at a time are:

- The drug goes directly into the bloodstream, quickly reaching the body part needing medication.
- The drug is delivered steadily over an extended period of time.

Uses for an IV include to replenish body fluids and to keep a vein open for future use.

Of great importance in IV use is the flow rate. The flow rate is an indication of how fast the fluid is entering the vein. Typical flow rates, called *microdrops*, are 60 drops per mL. A *macrodrop* may be 10, 15, or 20 drops per mL.

The standard notation for drops per mL is drop/mL. Consider, however, this notation: 120 drops/2 mL. The result should be the same as 60 drops/1 mL. But it could be argued that 60 drops cannot be divided by 2 mL—that we can divide only 120/2.

Nevertheless, it is convenient to treat dimensional symbols, such as drops and mL, much like variables. Compare, for example,

$$120x/2y = (120/2)(x/y) = 60(x/y)$$

to

$$120dr/2mL = (120/2)(dr/mL) = 60(dr/mL).$$

This analogy holds in other situations as well. For example, 2 feet + 3 meters compares to $2x + 3y$.

What Do You Think?

"I don't want students working on me." You are in your final year of training. The census is very high at the hospital where you are practicing. As luck would have it, among the patients on whom you are working this morning is Mrs. Smith—the woman who refuses to allow students to work on her. "If I'm paying these ridiculous prices, I want somebody who has graduated and who knows what they're doing. I'm not paying good money to have someone practice on me."

There is a distinct possibility that you will not be able to "trade" Mrs. Smith for another patient. How are you going to handle this? Do you need to consider any ethical or legal issues?

CHAPTER **18**

An Introduction to Equations

ADDITIONAL QUESTIONS

1. An equation is a statement that two quantities are _____.

2. Some equations can be solved by subtracting the _____ number from both sides of the equation.

3. Variable substitutions that make equations true are called _____.

4. Determine whether each of the following is a solution for the given equation.

   a. 2 for the equation $3x + 5 = 11$ _____

   b. −1 for the equation $2(x + 3) = 4$ _____

   c. 10 for the equation $x/2 − 3 = 2$ _____

   d. 3 for the equation $2(y + 1) = 3y + 2$ _____

5. Solve each of the following equations.

   a. $3x = 15$ _____

   b. $y + 6 = 9$ _____

   c. $3x + 1 = 10$ _____

   d. $2p − 6 = 4$ _____

   e. $3x/2 = −6$ _____

   f. $6x + 1 = 5x + 2$ _____

   g. $2 − 3y = y + 1$ _____

   h. $2(a + 2) = 3(4 − a)$ _____

6. Using the formula in your textbook, what is the ideal body weight (IBW) of a 5′6″ female? _____

7. Plastic has a density of 1.7 grams/cc and a volume of 3.5 cc. Use the formula $m = dv$ to find its mass.

   _____

   _____

8. Rewrite the formula in the previous problem to find the density of an object with a mass of 7 grams and a volume of 3.2 cc.

   _____

   _____

9. Find the HR (in bpm) for 55 HB in 20 seconds.

_____

_____

10. Find the MAP for a systolic pressure of 150 mm Hg and a diastolic pressure of 60 mm Hg.

_____

_____

ADDITIONAL ACTIVITIES/LABS

1. This activity will visually demonstrate balancing equations. Borrow some balance scales from the science department of your school. After your teacher divides the class into groups, use paper clips to demonstrate the use of the balance scale. Ask one person in the group to put a secret number of paper clips in an envelope, close the envelope, and put it along with some additional clips into pan one. The remaining students should add one envelope, and then one clip at a time, to pan two until the pans balance. Write an equation to represent the result. For example, if there were 3 extra clips in pan one, with the sealed envelope, and 8 clips in pan two, the equation could be written $x + 3 = 8$. Next, remove one clip at a time from each side, realizing that the pans still balance, to get the result of the equation for our previous example, $x = 5$.

2. Work with a partner to translate mathematical sentences into English. Use synonyms, such as "minus" and "less."

Extended Concepts

Factors That Control Blood Pressure

In order to control blood pressure (BP), it is important to understand the factors that determine blood pressure. The two primary factors are cardiac output (CO) and peripheral resistance (PR).

Cardiac output is the amount of blood pumped by the heart. The two factors that make up cardiac output are heart rate (HR) and stroke volume (SV). The formula for cardiac output is as follows:

$$CO = HR \times SV$$

Peripheral resistance is determined mainly by the diameter of the blood vessels. The overall formula for blood pressure can be written as follows:

$$BP = CO \times PR$$
$$BP = (HR \times SV) \times PR$$

If any of these three factors increase, blood pressure will also increase. Antihypertensive drugs lower blood pressure by decreasing cardiac output or reducing peripheral resistance.

Notice that using the concepts presented in this chapter, the formula could be changed, for example, to:

$$PR = \frac{BP}{(HR \times SV)}$$

This would allow the peripheral resistance to be found if the other variables are known.

What Do You Think?

The face of health care is changing. The traditional hospital is becoming more of an acute-care setting, and many of its services are offered at alternate sites. One such site is the patient's home. Patients, who previously may have spent more recovery time in the hospital, are now being discharged earlier, and more aggressive follow-up home care is given. What do you think about this? What are the advantages of home care? What are the disadvantages?

C H A P T E R **19**

More Equation Forms

ADDITIONAL QUESTIONS

1. What number is four more than 5? _____

2. Two-thirds of what number is five? _____

3. The area of Lake Superior is four times the area of Lake Ontario. If the area of Lake Superior is approximately 78,000 km, what is the area of Lake Ontario? _____

4. Ethyl alcohol boils at 78.3°C. This is 13.5°C more than the boiling point of methyl alcohol. What is the boiling point of methyl alcohol? _____

5. A doctor makes three times his salary of 10 years ago. If his current salary is $258,000, what was his salary 10 years ago? _____

6. Solve the following ratios:

   a. $v/15 = 120/180$ _____

   b. $16/t = 4/9$ _____

7. A pitcher gave up 71 runs in 285 innings. At this rate, how many runs did the pitcher give up each 9 innings? _____

8. To determine the number of fish in a lake, a biologist catches 255 fish, tags them, and throws them back in the lake. Later, 50 fish are caught, and 20 of them are found to be tagged. Estimate the number of fish in the lake. _____

9. A department uses 234 bottles of medication in 14 days. At the same ratio, how many bottles will the department need for a 42-day period? _____

10. If a drug is to be given 10 mg per kg of body weight, how much of the drug should be given to a 150-lb patient? _____

ADDITIONAL ACTIVITIES/LABS

1. Borrow some science books, especially physics and chemistry books, from your science department. Examine these texts, looking for formulas and where formulas are used. Write these on the board and solve for certain variables.

2. Given the following information, what should be the equation?

x	1	2	3	4
y	5	6	7	8

Invent a table that has a corresponding equation. Share this with a partner, and see whether your partner can either guess the equation or come up with an alternate equation that fits the table.

Extended Concepts

Variations

We are often interested not only in the formula for a given quantity, but also in the relationship between the formula variables. If two variables are related so that as one increases, the other also increases, we say that they are *directly proportional*. For example, if Q increases as P increases, we say that "Q is proportional to P." This means that as P increases or decreases, Q will do likewise. This could be written as the equation $Q = kP$, where k represents a constant value. Notice that if P were to double, Q would also double, which can be expressed as: $Q = k(2P)$ or $Q = 2kP$.

Poiseuille's law describes variation as it applies to the rate of flow of liquid through a tube. If Q represents how fast a liquid flows through a tube, and R represents the radius of the tube, Poiseuille's law (under controlled conditions) might be written, "Q is proportional to the fourth power of the radius of the tube," or, in equation form, $Q = kR^4$. This means that as the radius of the tube increases, the rate of flow of the liquid also increases. This seems reasonable; a larger tube would allow more liquid through. Notice, however, that Q is proportional to the fourth power of R. As R doubles, $Q = k(2R)^4$ or $16kR^4$, which is sixteen times larger. That is, if the radius of the tube doubles, the flow rate increases sixteen-fold.

Think of how this relates to the flow rate of blood through your arteries. If your arteries were to become clogged with plaque, and the radii were thus reduced by one-half, the flow rate would be reduced to one-sixteenth of its original rate. Poiseuille's law thus demonstrates why a buildup of plaque in the arteries can be so dangerous.

What Do You Think?

Skilled nursing home facilities are changing dramatically. Rather than sending geriatric patients having pneumonia to hospitals, some facilities are treating these patients on-site. Some argue that the level of care received in nursing home facilities is not as good as that received in hospitals. However, many nursing homes have hired higher-skilled personnel to treat patients in-house. What do you think? What are the advantages? What are the disadvantages?

C H A P T E R **20**

Statistics and Graphs

ADDITIONAL QUESTIONS

1. _____ is the branch of mathematics concerned with the collection, organization, and display of information. This information is referred to as _____.

2. The three measures of central tendency are _____, _____, and _____.

3. Nine patients had the following respective temperatures in degrees Fahrenheit: 97.3, 98.2, 98.8, 98.9, 99.0, 99.7, 100.0, 102.6, and 103.1. What are the mean, median, and mode for these temperatures? _____, _____, _____

4. A healthy female has a total daily caloric intake of approximately 2,200 calories. The following graph shows the recommended daily percentages of protein, fat, and carbohydrates.

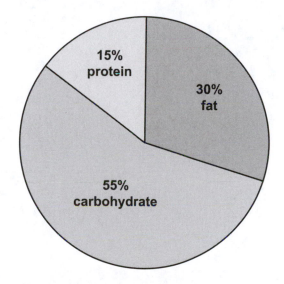

a. Approximately how many times more calories should come from carbohydrates than from protein? _____ from carbohydrates than from fat? _____

b. Given this woman's daily intake of 2,200 calories, find the recommended caloric intake for each of the following.

protein: _____   fat: _____   carbohydrates: _____

5. For a 12-month period from January to December, a department used the following number of bottles of saline solution (in order): 231, 265, 210, 250, 260, 280, 300, 310, 350, 260, 255, and 210.

   a. Draw a bar graph illustrating this information.

   b. According to your bar graph, during which three months were the most bottles of saline solution used? _____

   c. Draw a line graph using the same information.

   d. During which months were the fewest bottles of saline solution used? _____

   e. In light of the fact that saline solution can be used to help in cases of dehydration, explain how these numbers may make sense. _____

ADDITIONAL ACTIVITIES/LABS

1. Find data on some area of interest and construct a bulletin board that uses graphs to represent that data graphically.

2. After being separated into groups, collect data and represent it using a graph. For example, one group could determine how many students have each of a number of different colors of hair, and draw a bar graph representing this data. Another group could measure the heights of students to the nearest 5 inches, and represent this information via a bar graph.

3. Bring in graphs from newspapers and discuss the appropriateness of the graphs.

4. For two weeks, follow whether a stock on the New York Stock Exchange gains or loses. Draw a line graph of the results. Try to predict the next day's result.

Extended Concepts

Straight Line Depreciation

A hospital buys a machine for $520,000. The machine is expected to last for 8 years, at which time its trade-in, or scrap, value will be $130,000. Over its lifetime, the machine will depreciate $520,000 − $130,000, or $390,000. If hospital administration projects that this decline in value will be the same each year—that is, 1/8 of $390,000, or $48,750 per year—they are using what is called straight line depreciation. This is illustrated in the following graph.

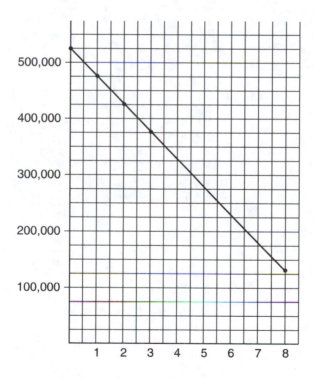

After one year, the value of the machine will be $520,000 − $48,750, or $471,250. After two years, the machine will be worth $471,250 − $48,750, or $422,500. The values for years three through eight ($337,500, $325,000, etc.) can also be read from the graph.

What Do You Think?

Statistics can be manipulated, or only select statistics reported. For example, a hospital survey may reveal that 80% of the patients surveyed on the obstetrics floor were satisfied with their stays. The hospital may then generalize and report that "the majority of our patients are happy with our services, and feel ours to be a good hospital." What is wrong with this conclusion?

Chemistry in the Health Sciences

C H A P T E R **21**

Energy and States of Matter

ADDITIONAL QUESTIONS

1. A can weighing 20 newtons is sitting on a shelf 6 meters above the floor. What is the potential energy of the can relative to the floor? _____

2. The can in question 1 fell to the floor. Neglecting friction, its velocity just prior to striking the floor was 11 m/sec. If it has a mass of 2 kg, what was its kinetic energy at this point? _____

3. A sample of mercury has a mass of 3,380 grams and occupies a volume of 250 milliliters. What is the density of mercury? _____

4. A patient's urine has a lower-than-normal specific gravity. What are some causes of a lower-than-normal specific gravity?

   _____

   _____

   _____

5. List several factors that will cause the specific gravity of urine to be higher than normal.

   _____

   _____

   _____

6. A woman weighing 110 pounds is walking in high-heeled shoes. Each shoe heel has an area of 1/16 square inch. Assuming that all of the woman's weight is on her heels at some point while she is walking, what pressure is she exerting on the pavement at that point? _____

7. Given the density of water is 64 lb/ft^3, what pressure would be exerted on a diver at a depth of 100 feet?

   _____

8. Refer to the figure below. What happens to the temperature as ice changes to water at 0°C? What happens to the energy applied to the system?

_____

_____

_____

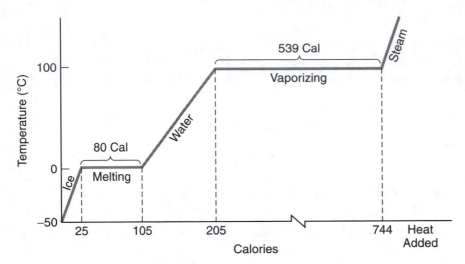

9. The energy possessed by a baseball as it travels from the pitcher to the catcher is called:

   a. potential energy

   b. stored energy

   c. heat energy

   d. kinetic energy

10. The physical state(s) of matter is(are):

    a. solid

    b. liquid

    c. gas

    d. all of the above

11. The state of matter in which the particles vibrate about a fixed point is called a(an):

    a. liquid

    b. gas

    c. solid

    d. plasma state

12. If the density of an object is less than the density of a gas or liquid in which it is immersed, it will:

    a. sink

    b. fly out of the liquid or gas

    c. float

    d. explode

13. Which of the following are units of pressure?

    a. pounds/square inch

    b. newtons/square meter

    c. pounds

    d. both a and b

14. The deeper you dive into a swimming pool, the pressure exerted on your body:

    a. remains the same

    b. decreases

    c. increases

    d. decreases and then increases

15. The principle that allows you to float a paper clip on water is:

    a. capillary action

    b. water pressure

    c. adhesive force

    d. surface tension

16. Thermal energy always moves from an object with a(an) _____ temperature to an object with a(an) _____ temperature.

    a. lower, higher

    b. lower, lower

    c. higher, higher

    d. higher, lower

17. The most common device for measuring temperature is a(an):

    a. thermometer

    b. bimetallic strip

    c. thermister

    d. thermocouple

18. The unit for measuring heat energy is the:

    a. Celsius unit

    b. calorie

    c. Kelvin unit

    d. newton

Matching 1

Match the following terms with their correct definition.

_____ 1. potential energy

_____ 2. kinetic energy

_____ 3. density

_____ 4. adhesive force

_____ 5. heat

a. mass per unit volume

b. energy of motion

c. transfer of heat energy from one body to another

d. stored energy

e. force of attraction

Matching 2

Match the following formulas with their correct definition.

_____ 1. mgh

_____ 2. ½(mv²)

_____ 3. m/v

_____ 4. f/a

_____ 5. D(h)

a. density (D)

b. kinetic energy (KE)

c. potential energy

d. pressure of a liquid (p)

e. pressure (p)

ADDITIONAL ACTIVITIES/LABS

1. Using a balance to determine mass and a graduated cylinder to measure volume, determine the density of several solids provided by your teacher.

2. Fill two 1-liter beakers with water. Place a can of diet soda in one beaker and a can of regular soda in the other beaker.

   Fill a beaker about half full of water. Fill another beaker about half full of rubbing alcohol. Place an ice cube into the beaker of water and another ice cube into the beaker of rubbing alcohol.

   Can you explain what happened in terms of density?

3. Carefully fill a glass of water so that the water surface is higher than the rim. Add a few drops of soap solution. What happens? Next fill another beaker half full of water. Place some pepper on the water. Some of the pepper should float. What happens to the floating pepper when you add a few drops of soap solution? Do you understand why some people say that soap makes water wetter?

4. Cut some paper towels into strips approximately 1 inch wide. Place a small drop of green food coloring approximately 1 inch from the bottom of a strip. Suspend the paper towel strip in a beaker containing approximately one-half inch of water, making sure that the food coloring spot does not come into contact with the water. What is the name of the process whereby the water moves up the paper?

5. Measure the temperature of boiling water. Does the temperature change while the water is boiling? What happens to the energy supplied to the boiling water?

Extended Concepts

The textbook defines absolute zero as the lowest temperature possible. This temperature is approximately $-273°C$. The lowest temperature ever recorded in the United States was $-62°C$, recorded in the state of Alaska in 1971. Scientists have not been able to achieve absolute zero in the laboratory. As noted in the text, temperature is the average kinetic energy of a substance. As the temperature of a substance approaches absolute zero, any slight vibration of the container holding the substance will impart kinetic energy to the substance particles and, hence, raise the temperature of the substance.

Unusual things happen to gases as they approach absolute zero. For example, helium will liquefy at a temperature of $-268.6°C$ (4.4 K). At a temperature below 2.1 K ($-270.9°C$), however, helium becomes a superfluid and has zero viscosity. The superfluid helium will actually flow up the sides and out of its container.

Other substances become superconductors at extremely low temperatures; that is, they have no resistance to electric currents flowing through them. If you were to start an electric current flowing through a loop of a semiconductor, the current would flow forever without diminishing. One application of superconductors is in the development of electromagnets. Physicists are currently trying to find superconducting materials that will work at higher temperatures.

What Do You Think?

From what you have learned thus far, why do you think body temperature is lowered for certain operations? Did you ever notice that hospital operating rooms are usually cool?

C H A P T E R **22**

Basic Concepts of Chemistry

ADDITIONAL QUESTIONS

1. Define the following terms:

   a. proton

   _____

   b. neutron

   _____

   c. electron

   _____

   d. nucleus

   _____

   e. atomic number

   _____

   f. mass number

   _____

2. An atom has 15 protons and 16 neutrons in its nucleus.

   a. What is its atomic number?   _____

   b. What is its mass number?   _____

   c. How many electrons surround the nucleus?   _____

3. Atoms of the same element but having different numbers of neutrons in their nucleus are
   called _____.

4. Find the group numbers of the following elements on the periodic table and write the symbol of the element.

	Group Number	Symbol
a. boron	_____	_____
b. iodine	_____	_____
c. calcium	_____	_____
d. sodium	_____	_____
e. carbon	_____	_____
f. sulfur	_____	_____

Periodic Table of the Elements[a]

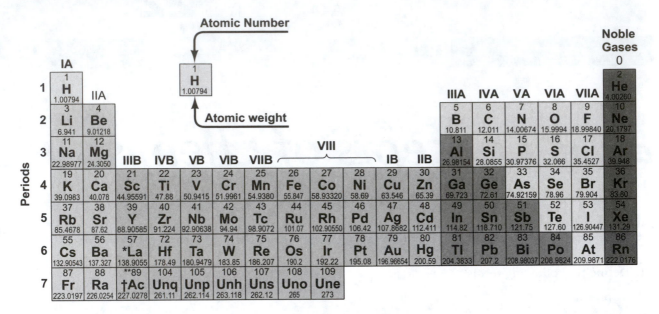

5. If X is used to represent the symbol of any element, what do *a* and *m* represent in the following symbol?

$$_aX^m$$

_____

_____

_____

6. Give the symbol, mass number, and charge for alpha, beta, and gamma radiation.

_____

_____

_____

7. Define the term *metastasis*.

_____

_____

_____

8. How does radon gas harm you?

_____

_____

_____

9. The symbol for the element sodium is:

   a. S

   b. So

   c. Na

   d. N

10. The subatomic particle that has a positive charge and a mass number of 1 is:

    a. proton

    b. neutron

    c. electron

    d. positron

11. The atomic number of an element is 10 and it has a mass number of 22. How many protons does it have in its nucleus?

    a. 22

    b. 10

    c. 12

    d. 2

12. An element has 13 protons and 14 neutrons. What is its mass number?

    a. 13

    b. 27

    c. 14

    d. 1

13. An element has an atomic number of 20 and a mass number of 41. How many electrons surround its nucleus?

    a. 21

    b. 42

    c. 61

    d. 20

14. The electron dot structure of sodium would be:

    a. Na

    b. Na:

    c. Na·

    d. :Na:

15. Iron is an important constituent of _____ in the blood.

    a. hemoglobin

    b. white blood cells

    c. leukocytes

    d. platelets

16. The radiation with the most penetrating power is:

    a. alpha

    b. beta

    c. positrons

    d. gamma

17. The radioisotope used to diagnose thyroid problems is:

    a. Iron-53

    b. Cobalt-60

    c. Technetium-99m

    d. Iodine-121

18. The imaging technique that doesn't use ionizing radiation is a(an):

    a. X-ray

    b. CAT scan

    c. MRI

    d. PET scan

Matching 1

Match the following symbols with the correct name of the element.

_____	1. sodium	a. K
_____	2. chlorine	b. Mg
_____	3. oxygen	c. Na
_____	4. potassium	d. O
_____	5. calcium	e. Cl
_____	6. hydrogen	f. Ca
_____	7. nitrogen	g. H
_____	8. magnesium	h. N

Matching 2

Match the correct definition with the following imaging techniques.

_____	1. X-ray	a. uses X-rays to produce a cross-sectional image of the body
_____	2. CAT scan	b. uses a strong magnetic field and radio waves to produce image
_____	3. MRI	c. uses high-energy electromagnetic radiation to produce image
_____	4. PET scan	d. uses an electron with a positive charge to produce image

ADDITIONAL ACTIVITIES/LABS

1. Observe the display of various elements as set up by your teacher. Gather the following information for each element in the display and organize the information in a table format.

   Symbol

   Atomic number

   Observations

   Metal or nonmetal

2. Use a Geiger counter to test various household items such as a smoke detector, mantles from a gas lantern, and old watches with luminous dials. See if you can detect any radiation.

Extended Concepts

In this chapter, we discussed some of the elements that are essential to proper health. Two of them, iron and copper, are needed in only extremely small amounts. We call these types of elements *trace elements*. Many other trace elements are needed by the body. While the amounts needed by the body have been well established for some trace elements, the daily requirement for others is unknown. In other cases, researchers know that a compound is needed by the body, but they do no not know exactly what role the compound plays in the body.

One of the more important trace elements is copper. Copper is found in shellfish, dried peas and beans, and chocolate. Copper is a component of many enzymes of the body, one of which helps in the formation of blood vessels, tendons, and bones. The daily requirement for copper is approximately 3×10^{-6} g, a-n extremely small amount.

Zinc is a trace element important in fetal development and nutrition of infants. In addition, zinc plays a role in carbohydrate, lipid, and protein metabolism. The best sources of zinc are protein-rich foods.

Some other trace elements, along with the diseases that a lack of these elements cause, are as follows: cobalt, pernicious anemia; manganese, convulsive disorders; selenium, Keshan disease; chromium, which plays a role in lowering blood sugar.

As you can see, the body requires many different elements in order to function properly, and these elements are not all found in any one source. It is necessary, therefore, to eat a variety of foods to obtain the essential elements needed by the body.

What Do You Think?

After you become a health care professional, continuing education is critically important. Rapid changes in knowledge, skills, diagnostics, and therapies demand a commitment to continuing health care education. How can an organization facilitate this? How can it ensure the same level of education to personnel who work the "off shifts" such as 3:00 P.M. to 11:00 P.M. or 11:00 P.M. to 7:00 A.M.? What incentives can be provided to encourage participation in a continuing health care education program?

C H A P T E R **23**

Bonding and Chemical Formulas

ADDITIONAL QUESTIONS

1. When a sodium atom loses an electron, the resulting ion will have a _____ charge.

2. When a sulfur atom gains two electrons, the resulting ion will have a _____ charge.

3. The movement of water through a cell membrane from a lower concentration of dissolved substances to a higher concentration of dissolved substances is called _____.

4. What is the difference between a pure covalent bond and a polar covalent bond?

   _____

   _____

   _____

5. Define the term *hydrogen bond*.

   _____

   _____

   _____

6. Write the symbol and charge for each of the following ions.

   a. lithium   _____

   b. aluminum   _____

   c. sulfate   _____

   d. bromide   _____

7. Name the following ions.

   a. S^{-2} _____

   b. F^{-1} _____

   c. Cu^{2+} _____

   d. $PO_4{}^{3-}$ _____

8. Write the formula for each of the following compounds.

   a. copper II chloride   _____

   b. sodium nitrate   _____

   c. calcium phosphate   _____

   d. sodium chloride   _____

9. Name the following compounds.

   a. $Al_2(SO_4)_3$ _____

   b. $Ca(OH)_2$ _____

   c. $Mg(NO_3)_2$ _____

   d. FeS   _____

10. The Avogadro number is _____.

11. Write a balanced formula equation for each of the following reactions.

    a. sodium hydroxide + hydrogen chloride → sodium chloride + water

    _____

    b. calcium nitrate + sodium phosphate → calcium phosphate + sodium nitrate

    _____

12. Balance the following equations.

    a. $H_2 + O_2 \rightarrow H_2O$ _____

    b. $Mg + HCl \rightarrow MgCl_2 + H_2$ _____

13. Which of the following is not a symptom of hypocalcemia?

    a. cardiac arrhythmia

    b. muscle twitching

    c. anorexia

    d. tetany

14. A solution that has the same concentration as the body's cells is said to be _____ relative to the body's cells.

    a. hypertonic

    b. isotonic

    c. hypotonic

    d. atonic

15. A solution with a concentration of 10.2% is said to be _____ relative to physiological saline solution.

    a. isotonic

    b. hypotonic

    c. atonic

    d. hypertonic

16. The type of bonding that results from the equal sharing of electrons is called:

    a. pure covalent bonding

    b. ionic bonding

    c. hydrogen bonding

    d. polar covalent bonding

17. The molecular formula for rubbing alcohol is C_3H_8O. How many oxygen atoms are in isopropyl alcohol?

    a. 0

    b. 1

    c. 3

    d. 8

18. The symbol and charge for the oxide ion is:

    a. Ox^{2-}

    b. O

    c. O^{2-}

    d. O^-

19. The formula for the compound magnesium chloride is:

    a. MgCl

    b. $MgCl_2$

    c. MaC

    d. $MaCl_2$

20. The type of bond that results from the unequal sharing of electrons is called _____ bonding.

    a. ionic

    b. pure covalent

    c. polar covalent

    d. hydrogen

21. When the equation $N_2 + H_2 \rightarrow NH_3$ is correctly balanced, the coefficient in front of H_2 is:

    a. 0

    b. 1

    c. 2

    d. 3

22. The balanced formula equation for the word equation hydrogen plus oxygen yields water is:

    a. $2H + O \rightarrow H_2O$

    b. $2H_2 + O_2 \rightarrow 2H_2O$

    c. $H + O \rightarrow HO$

    d. $H_2 + O_2 \rightarrow H_2O$

Matching 1

Match the following names of ions with their correct symbols.

_____ 1. chloride

_____ 2. potassium

_____ 3. calcium

_____ 4. iodide

_____ 5. sulfide

_____ 6. sodium

a. K^+

b. Cl^-

c. S^{2-}

d. I^-

e. Na^+

f. Ca^{2+}

Matching 2

Match the following formulas of compounds to their correct names.

_____ 1. $CaCl_2$

_____ 2. $NaHCO_3$

_____ 3. K_2SO_4

_____ 4. $Mg_3(PO_4)_2$

_____ 5. $CaHPO_4$

_____ 6. $FeSO_4$

a. calcium chloride

b. magnesium phosphate

c. iron II sulfate

d. potassium sulfate

e. sodium bicarbonate

f. calcium monohydrogen phosphate

ADDITIONAL ACTIVITIES/LABS

1. Use a conductivity meter to determine whether various solutions, as provided by your teacher, are electrolytes or nonelectrolytes.

2. Fill a clean 250-mL beaker half full with demineralized water. Place 1 milliliter of the water from the beaker in the well of a spot plate and add several drops of 1 M silver nitrate. A white precipitate indicates the presence of chloride ions.

   Next, test a solution of 1% sodium chloride for chloride ions, as described previously. Obtain a 15-cm length of dialyzing membrane and moisten in distilled water. Make clean holes in each end so that the membrane can eventually be supported in a beaker as shown in the following figure. Using a funnel, place approximately 20 milliliters of sodium chloride solution into the dialyzing membrane, being careful not to contaminate the outside of the membrane. Suspend the system in the 250-mL beaker for approximately a half an hour. After this time, test the water in the beaker for chloride ions.

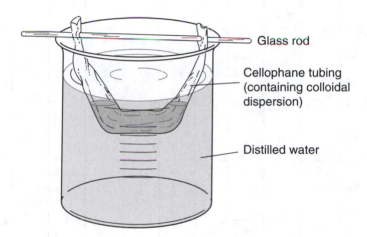

   Glass rod

   Cellophane tubing
   (containing colloidal
   dispersion)

   Distilled water

3. Memorize the symbols and charges of the ions in Tables 23-2 and 23-3 of the text. After your teacher divides the class into two equal groups, conduct a "spelling bee" wherein contestants must give the symbol and charge for a given ion.

4. Obtain two iron nails and use sandpaper to shine them. Place one of the nails in water in a way that it is partially exposed to the air and place the other nail on the desk. Observe what happens to the nails during the week. Water is a catalyst for rusting.

Extended Concepts

In this chapter, we discussed some of the ions, or electrolytes, that are necessary for the body to function properly. However, we did not specify where these ions are found. The blood plasma, interstitial fluid, and cellular fluid are among the places where electrolytes are found in the body. (Interstitial fluid is found in tissues but not in the blood or in cells.)

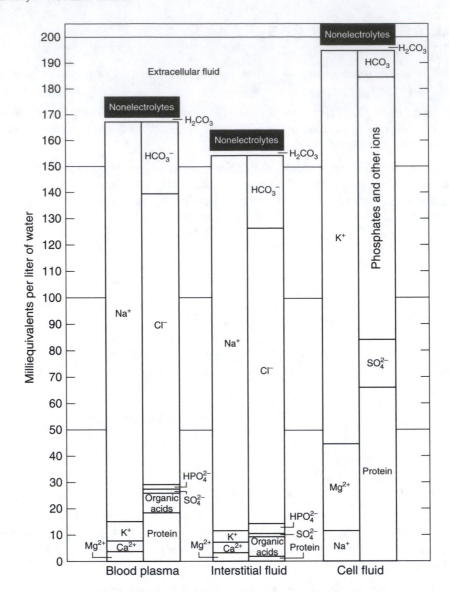

The above figure shows the electrolyte compositions of blood plasma, interstitial fluid, and cellular fluid. As illustrated in the figure Na^+, Cl^-, and HCO_3^- are the major components of the blood. The electrolyte composition of interstitial fluid is similar to that of blood. The electrolyte composition of cellular fluid, however, is quite different from that of blood or interstitial fluid. The most abundant positive ions are K^+ and Mg^{2+}, whereas phosphate and other ions constitute the major negative ions in cells. Beverages such as Gatorade are used to replenish these electrolytes, which are lost whenever a person exercises.

What Do You Think?

Malpractice and Negligence

The terms *malpractice* (*mal* meaning bad) and *negligence* are often used as synonyms. There is a difference between the two, however. Negligence means not doing something that a reasonable man or woman should do in a certain situation. Any individual can be negligent, for example, the individual who recklessly drives a car and injures another person as a result. Only a professional person such as a health care practitioner, however, can commit malpractice. Malpractice can result from lack of skill, failure to render service, failure to maintain currency in knowledge or technique, or practices that are evil, immoral, or illegal. Can you think of ways to prevent or minimize malpractice occurrences?

Quality of Life

Whether by tragic accident, disease state, or severe birth defect, the question may arise whether someone should receive medical treatment to sustain a life that has no "quality."

The term *quality of life* is very vague and is used in a number of ways depending on who is making the judgment and what standards are being applied. Some judgments are based on the patient's own values and preferences. For example, a patient may state that if advanced life-support systems are required to sustain life, death is preferred.

In other circumstances, others may be making such judgments for the patient and thus rely on their own sets of values rather than on the patient's. What would be your considerations should you need to give input regarding whether to withhold extraordinary medical treatment from an individual based on a quality-of-life judgment? How do you define your quality of life? Under what circumstances would you not want extraordinary means used to keep you alive?

Name: _____   Date: _____

CHAPTER **24**

The Gas Laws

ADDITIONAL QUESTIONS

1. What are three postulates of the kinetic theory?

   _____

   _____

   _____

2. _____ _____ states that at a given temperature and pressure, equal volumes of all gases contain equal numbers of molecules.

3. Absolute zero on the Celsius temperature scale is _____.

4. A temperature of −70°C is equivalent to what Kelvin temperature? _____

5. State Boyle's law.

   _____

   _____

   _____

6. What law states that if the mass and pressure of a gas remain constant, volume and temperature of the gas are directly related? _____

7. If nitrogen makes up approximately 78% of the air, and the air pressure is 710 mm Hg, what is the partial pressure of nitrogen? _____

8. State Henry's law.

   _____

   _____

   _____

9. Why does a bottle of soda fizz when it is opened?

   _____

   _____

   _____

10. What are three factors that affect the rate of a reaction?

    _____

    _____

    _____

11. Why shouldn't you take an antipyretic if your temperature is less than 101°F?

_____

_____

_____

12. _____ is a condition in which the body temperature is lower than normal.

13. What happens to the average kinetic energy of a substance if its temperature is increased?

_____

_____

_____

14. Which of the following is not a postulate of the kinetic theory of gases?

    a. Matter is composed of very small particles.

    b. Equal volumes of all gases contain the same number of particles.

    c. The particles of a gas are in constant motion.

    d. The particles of the gas undergo elastic collisions.

15. If the absolute temperature of a gas decreases, the average velocity of the gas particles will:

    a. decrease

    b. increase

    c. remain the same

16. If the pressure exerted on a gas is doubled, the volume at constant temperature will:

    a. double

    b. increase

    c. decrease

    d. decrease by one half

17. If the temperature of a gas is increased at constant pressure, the volume will:

    a. decrease

    b. remain the same

    c. increase

18. At constant volume, if the temperature of a gas is increased, the pressure will:

    a. remain the same

    b. decrease

    c. increase

19. The following gases are mixed in a container. What is the total pressure of the mixture?
    N_2 = 150 mm Hg, O_2 = 100 mm Hg, and Ar = 200 mm Hg

    a. 450 mm Hg

    b. 200 mm Hg

    c. 100 mm Hg

20. STPD stands for:

    a. safe temperature, pressure, and dry

    b. standard temperature, plain, and dry

    c. standard temperature, pressure, and dry

    d. safe temperature, plain, and dry

21. _____ is the movement of a gas from an area of high concentration of the gas to an area of low concentration.

    a. Diffusion

    b. Pressure

    c. Temperature

    d. Distillation

22. According to the collision theory, what two conditions are necessary for a chemical reaction to take place?

    a. proper temperature and correct pressure

    b. proper orientation of the molecules and sufficient energy

    c. proper orientation and correct pressure

    d. proper volume and sufficient energy

23. Which of the following is not a factor affecting the rate of a reaction?

    a. temperature

    b. humidity

    c. concentration

    d. presence catalysts

24. Match the following equations with the corresponding gas law.

    ____ 1. $\dfrac{V_1}{T_1} = \dfrac{V_2}{T_2}$ a. Charles' law

    ____ 2. $P_1V_1 = P_2V_2$ b. combined gas law

    ____ 3. $\dfrac{P_1}{T_1} = \dfrac{P_2}{T_2}$ c. Boyle's law

    ____ 4. $\dfrac{P_1 V_1}{T_1} = \dfrac{P_2 V_2}{T_2}$ d. Gay-Lussac's law

25. Match the following terms with their definitions.

    ____ 1. Avogadro's law   a. the amount of gas that dissolves in a solution is directly proportional to the partial pressure of the gas above the liquid

    ____ 2. absolute humidity   b. a substance that reduces fevers

    ____ 3. Henry's law   c. the minimum energy for a reaction to occur

    ____ 4. activation energy   d. at a given temperature and pressure, equal volumes of gases contain the same number of particles

    ____ 5. catalyst   e. actual weight of water vapor contained in a given amount of gas

    ____ 6. antipyretic   f. a substance that increases the rate of a reaction without being consumed

ADDITIONAL ACTIVITIES/LABS

1. Obtain a capillary tube that is open at one end and closed at the other. Use an eye dropper with a long, thin point to insert a drop of water about halfway down the tube, trapping some air in the closed end of the tube. Use a wax pencil to mark the level of the water. Insert the closed end of the capillary tube into some ice water in a beaker and note any changes. Then place the closed end of the capillary tube into a beaker of hot water and note any changes. Are your results consistent with Charles' law?

2. Partially blow up a small balloon and place it in a stoppered filter flask. Attach one end of vacuum to the flask and the other to an aspirator. Turn on the aspirator and observe what happens to the balloon. Are the results consistent with Boyle's law?

3. Place some soda from a freshly opened can into a stoppered filtering flask. Attach one end of a piece of vacuum hose to the flask and the other end to an aspirator. Turn on the water to the aspirator and observe. Can you explain what happened in terms of Henry's law?

4. Place a carrot in a saturated salt solution and observe what happens over the next several days. Explain your observations in terms of diffusion.

5. Draw a picture showing the boiling point of water, the freezing point of water, and absolute zero on the Fahrenheit, Celsius, and Kelvin temperature scales.

6. Prepare a beaker of ice water and a beaker of near boiling water. Obtain two light sticks and activate them. Place one of the light sticks in the hot water and one in cold water. After a few minutes, take the light sticks and observe which is brighter. Explain your observations.

Extended Concepts

Process of Breathing
This chapter examined the process of breathing. You should remember from your reading that in order to inhale, you must lower the pressure inside your chest cavity. The pressure inside the chest cavity being lower than the outside air pressure causes air to rush into your lungs. The act is no problem under normal circumstances. If the chest cavity were to be punctured by a gunshot or sharp object, however, it would be difficult to maintain the pressure difference. In fact, the lung might collapse because of the puncture wound. First aid in such a case would involve sealing the hole in some manner as to maintain the necessary pressure difference.

Direction of Reaction
As noted in the text, a simplified equation for the combining of oxygen and hemoglobin is $Hb + O_2 \rightleftharpoons HbO_2$. The double arrows indicate that this reaction is reversible, that is, it can go from left to right or right to left. How do you determine the direction of the reaction? It is determined by the concentrations. As explained in the text, the rate of reaction depends on concentration. Therefore, if the concentration of one of the substances involved in a reaction increases, that substance will dictate the direction of the reaction. This can be illustrated by considering a simplified version of what happens to hemoglobin as it travels in the bloodstream. In the lungs, the concentration of oxygen is relatively high. Thus, the reaction proceeds from left to right, that is, the oxygenation of hemoglobin is favored. At the cells, however, the oxygen concentration is low, and the concentration of oxygenated hemoglobin (HbO_2) is high. Therefore, the reaction is favored from right to left, and oxygen is released.

What Do You Think?
Communication is an extremely important characteristic of a quality allied health care provider. This is true whether you are communicating with patients, physicians, other allied health personnel, or nurses. List and discuss those attributes that make a good communicator.

Name: _____ Date: _____

C H A P T E R **25**

Acids and Bases

ADDITIONAL QUESTIONS

1. A(an) _____ is a proton acceptor.

2. The formula for the hydronium ion is _____.

3. As the hydrogen ion concentration in a solution increases, the hydroxide ion concentration _____.

4. A(an) _____ is an ionic substance formed from the positive ion of a base and a negative ion of an acid.

5. When the pH of blood falls below 7.35, a condition called _____ exists.

6. _____ solutions have the ability to neutralize acids and bases within certain limits and thereby maintain a constant pH.

7. The lungs help neutralize hydrogen ions in the blood by removing _____ _____ from the body.

8. The brain can regulate hydrogen ion concentration in the blood by increasing or decreasing the _____ rate.

9. The muscle pain and cramping we experience due to overexertion is caused by _____.

10. Which of the following is not a property of an acid?

    a. dissolves metals

    b. neutralizes bases

    c. tastes bitter

    d. turns litmus red

11. Which of the following is not a property of a base?

    a. neutralizes acids

    b. is caustic

    c. turns litmus blue

    d. tastes sour

12. The acid found in the stomach is called:

    a. hydrochloric acid

    b. acetic acid

    c. sulfuric acid

    d. vinegar

13. Which of the following is the pH of an acid?

    a. 7.0

    b. 8.0

    c. 6.5

    d. 10

14. A blood pH below 7.35 is referred to as:

    a. normal

    b. an acid solution

    c. alkalosis

    d. acidosis

15. The main buffer in the blood is the _____ buffer.

    a. bicarbonate

    b. hydrochlorate

    c. phosphate

    d. protein

16. The lungs help to maintain the proper pH of the blood by removing:

    a. water vapor

    b. oxygen

    c. carbon dioxide

    d. nitrogen

17. The kidneys help to maintain the proper pH of the blood by maintaining proper amounts of _____ in the blood.

    a. water

    b. oxygen

    c. phosphate ion

    d. bicarbonate ion

18. Breaking down glucose without oxygen is called:

    a. aerobic metabolism

    b. fat metabolism

    c. anaerobic metabolism

    d. glucogenesis

19. Carbonic acid (H_2CO_3) yields _____ when it decomposes.

    a. H^+ and CO_3^{2-}

    b. H_2O and CO_2

    c. H, C, and O

    d. H_2 and CO_2

20. Match the following terms with their correct definition.

    ____ 1. acid

    ____ 2. base

    ____ 3. caustic

    ____ 4. pH

    ____ 5. acidosis

    ____ 6. buffer solution

    a. dissolves animal tissue

    b. a blood pH less than 7.35

    c. a solution that maintains a relatively constant pH

    d. a proton donor

    e. a proton acceptor

    f. a measure of acid concentration

21. Match the following pHs with the proper term in the second column.

    ____ 1. 8.5

    ____ 2. 2.5

    ____ 3. 1.0

    ____ 4. 7.0

    ____ 5. 6.5

    a. acid

    b. base

    c. neutral

ADDITIONAL ACTIVITIES/LABS

1. Using universal pH test paper, test the pHs of some solutions. Test solutions from your laboratory as well as some common household solutions.

2. Add 20 drops of 0.1 M HCl to a small evaporating dish. Add 20 drops of 0.1 M NaOH to this. Stir well and measure the pH. What was the pH value? What should it have been? Evaporate the solution to dryness. Can you identify the solid in the dish? The equation for the reaction is:

$$NaOH + HCl \rightarrow NaCl + H_2O$$

3. Prepare a phosphate buffer by thoroughly mixing 10 milliliters of 0.1 M Na_2HPO_4 with 10 milliliters of 0.1 M NaH_2PO_4 in a 50-mL beaker. Add 20 drops of universal indicator. Observe and record the color of the solution. Put 20 milliliters of boiled distilled water into a 50-mL beaker. Add 20 drops of universal indicator and note the color.

    Add two drops of 0.5 M HCl to both the phosphate buffer and the boiled distilled water. Observe the colors and record the pHs. In which case did the pH change the most?

Extended Concepts

As noted in the text, the lungs play a role in controlling the pH of the blood. In cases where the lungs are not functioning properly, acidosis or alkalosis can develop. (Because the cause of such conditions is respiratory in nature, we refer to them as respiratory acidosis or respiratory alkalosis.)

For example, patients having severe emphysema involuntarily retain CO_2. As mentioned in the text, retaining CO_2 increases hydrogen ion concentration, resulting in respiratory acidosis. Other causes of respiratory acidosis include severe pneumonia, asthma, overdose of a depressant, and severe head injury. In fact, anything that decreases the rate at which CO_2 is eliminated from the body can cause respiratory acidosis.

On the other hand, anything that increases the rate at which CO_2 is eliminated from the body can cause respiratory alkalosis. For example, hysterics, rapid breathing at high altitude, disease of the central nervous system, or improper management of a ventilator will all increase the CO_2 elimination rate.

What Do You Think?

You have likely heard of employees who have "walked out" or are "on strike." Striking, as defined by Dorothy D. Nayer, is "an exercise of just, lawful, and ethical rights to withhold or withdraw labor in order to gain concessions from employers." What are your views regarding health professionals striking? Should health care workers be allowed to exercise this right? How would this conflict with their dedication to serve? What about the dangers to the public?

C H A P T E R **26**

Biochemistry

ADDITIONAL QUESTIONS

1. _____ are compounds having the same molecular formula but different structural formulas.

2. What is the structural difference between an alkane and an alkene?

   _____

   _____

   _____

3. How do monosaccharides, disaccharides, and polysaccharides differ?

   _____

   _____

   _____

4. A person having a blood sugar level of 50 mg/100 mL would be classified as _____.

5. The most abundant polysaccharide, which is undigestible by humans, is _____.

6. What is the structural difference between a saponifiable lipid and a nonsaponifiable lipid?

   _____

   _____

   _____

7. Distinguish between a saturated fatty acid and an unsaturated fatty acid.

   _____

   _____

   _____

8. Which of the following is not a property of organic compounds?

   a. Organic compounds don't dissolve in water.

   b. Organic compounds are more easily decomposed by heat.

   c. Organic compounds react at a slower rate.

   d. Organic substances dissolve in polar liquids.

9. Hydrocarbons with one or more double covalent bonds are called:

    a. alkenes

    b. alkanes

    c. alkynes

    d. carbohydrates

10. Which of the following is not an organic compound?

    a. CH_4

    b. NaCl

    c. CH_3CH_3

    d. CH_3CH_2OH

11. A _____ consists of two sugar molecules bonded together.

    a. polysaccharide

    b. monosaccharide

    c. disaccharide

    d. lipid

12. A blood sugar level of 150 mg/100 mL would be classified as:

    a. normal

    b. hypoglycemic

    c. hyperglycemic

13. The rarest blood type is:

    a. A

    b. AB

    c. O

    d. B

14. The hydrolysis of sucrose produces:

    a. 2 glucose

    b. glucose and maltose

    c. glucose and galactose

    d. glucose and fructose

15. The storage form of glucose in plants is called:

    a. starch

    b. disaccharide

    c. glycogen

    d. sucrose

16. Plant or animal substances that are soluble in nonpolar solvents are called:

    a. lipids

    b. proteins

    c. carbohydrates

    d. hormones

17. Organic acids and alcohols react to form which of these?

    a. carbohydrates

    b. lipids

    c. proteins

    d. disaccharides

18. Match the following alkanes with their correct name.

    ____ 1. CH_3CH_3 a. methane

    ____ 2. $CH_3CH_2CH_3$ b. ethane

    ____ 3. CH_4 c. pentane

    ____ 4. $CH_3CH_2CH_2CH_2CH_3$ d. butane

    ____ 5. $CH_3CH_2CH_2CH_3$ e. propane

19. Match the following terms with their correct definition.

    ____ 1. isomer   a. sugars and starches

    ____ 2. carbohydrate   b. lower-than-normal blood sugar level

    ____ 3. hypoglycemia   c. same molecular formula but different structural formula

    ____ 4. lipids   d. a hydrocarbon with an OH group attached

    ____ 5. alcohol   e. fats and oils

ADDITIONAL ACTIVITIES/LABS

1. Using molecular model kits, build models of the first three members of the alkane and alkene families. Draw structural formulas and name the first three members for both families.

2. Build a model of glucose and draw the structural formula of the molecule.

3. Use an iodine solution provided by your teacher to test several types of food for starch.

Extended Concepts

There has been much interest lately in omega-3 fatty acids. The interest in these compounds came about after a study revealed a low incidence of heart disease in Eskimos despite a high intake of fat, mainly from fish oils. Some scientists felt that high levels of omega-3 fatty acids present in fish oil provided protection against heart disease. Linolenic acid (Table 26-2 in the text) is an example of an omega-3 fatty acid. The name *omega-3* is derived from the carbon-carbon double bond being on the third carbon from the end of the hydrocarbon chain, as in linolenic acid. Linolenic acid is found in plant seed oils such as the oil from sunflower seeds. One of the acids found in fish is eicosapentaenoic acid (EPA). Both of these omega-3 fatty acids are believed to reduce the ability of platelets to stick together; that is, they inhibit blood clot formation. However, EPA is the more active inhibitor.

What Do You Think?

A major lawsuit can be not only financially difficult for a health care organization, but also harm the organization's reputation and image and, thus, cause decline in future business. Within each health care organization, therefore, a risk management office can usually be found. The goal of risk management is to prevent financial loss resulting from legal action. Risk management personnel attempt to identify, track, and correct any risks that could potentially cause financial loss. Such risks include loss of life via accidents, surgical error, malpractice, and lack of building maintenance, among other things. What are some areas of risk that you would be concerned about in a health care organization? How would you identify potential problems?

C H A P T E R **27**

The Amazing Proteins

ADDITIONAL QUESTIONS

1. The word *protein* is derived from the Greek word *proteios*, which means _____.

2. The building blocks of proteins are _____ _____.

3. Define the term *essential amino acid*.

   _____

   _____

   _____

4. Distinguish between a complete protein and an incomplete protein.

   _____

   _____

   _____

5. _____ is the disorganization of the protein structure in such a manner as to render the protein incapable of performing its function.

6. What is the difference between a globular protein and a fibrous protein?

   _____

   _____

   _____

7. List two classes of fibrous proteins. _____ _____

8. Which of the following is not a function of the proteins in the body?

   a. component of skin, hair, and cartilage

   b. component of muscles in our bodies

   c. transport oxygen and lipids in the bloodstream

   d. component of glycogen

9. Which of the following is an incomplete protein?

   a. fish

   b. beans

   c. egg

   d. meat

10. The process by which proteins are broken down into amino acids is called:

    a. hydrolysis

    b. denaturation

    c. deamination

    d. saponification

11. Which of the following is not a denaturing agent?

    a. heat

    b. violent whipping

    c. strong acids

    d. all of the above

12. Which of the following is a protein classification according to biological function?

    a. fibrous proteins

    b. globular proteins

    c. glycoproteins

    d. enzyme

13. Enzymes cause reaction rates to:

    a. increase

    b. decrease

    c. remain the same

14. The purely protein part of an enzyme is called the:

    a. apoenzyme

    b. cofactor

    c. coenzyme

    d. substrate

15. The inactive form of an enzyme is called a(an):

    a. cofactor

    b. apoenzyme

    c. zymogen

    d. substrate

16. The theory that only a substrate with a structure complementary to the structure of a given enzyme can bind with that enzyme is a statement of the:

    a. lock-and-key theory

    b. enzyme specificity theory

    c. enzyme substrate binding theory

    d. induced-fit theory

17. An enzyme that can be used to treat a heart attack is:

    a. CK, creatine kinase

    b. GOT, glutamate oxaloacetate aminotransferase

    c. LDH, lactate dehydrogenase

    d. TPA, tissue plasminogen activator

18. Match the following protein classifications according to biological function with their correct definition.

    _____ 1. enzymes

    _____ 2. hormones/neurotransmitters

    _____ 3. protection proteins

    _____ 4. structural proteins

    _____ 5. transport proteins

    a. carry other molecules in cells and blood

    b. catalysts within the body

    c. serve as major components of connective tissue

    d. chemical messengers within the body

    e. defend the body against disease

19. Match the following terms with their correct definitions.

    _____ 1. amino acids

    _____ 2. denaturation

    _____ 3. globular protein

    _____ 4. substrate

    _____ 5. coenzymes

    a. an organic cofactor

    b. spherical-shaped molecules that are water soluble

    c. disorganization of the protein structure

    d. building blocks of proteins

    e. substance acted on by an enzyme

ADDITIONAL ACTIVITIES/LABS

1. Draw condensed structural formulas for the following amino acids:

   a. glycine

   b. alanine

   c. serine

   d. cysteine

2. Using Figures 27-4 and 27-6 in the text, construct a model of an enzyme using cutouts from a sheet of paper. Identify the apoenzyme, cofactor, and active catalytic site. Construct a substrate that is compatible with the active catalytic site of the enzyme you prepared. Use these models to demonstrate the basics of enzyme action.

Extended Concepts

Have you or someone you know ever gone to a hairdresser for a permanent wave? You probably never considered the chemical reactions involved in the process of a permanent wave. But before discussing these reactions, it is important to consider some background information regarding proteins.

For a protein to function, it must maintain a particular shape. A protein maintains its shape via various types of attractive forces such as hydrogen bonding and the attraction between oppositely charged particles. Another such force is a covalent bond between sulfur atoms on different parts of the amino acid side chain. We refer to these interactions as disulfide links. The resulting forces between strands of amino acids help give the protein a particular three-dimensional shape. Denaturation of a protein causes the protein to lose its shape by interfering with these attractive forces.

A permanent wave concentrates on one of these forces—the disulfide link. During the first part of the permanent wave process, a reducing agent such as ammonium thioglycolate is used to treat the hair. This compound breaks the disulfide links. The hair is then put in curlers to yield the desired shape, and a different compound, such as potassium bromate or hydrogen peroxide, is applied to form new disulfide links within the hair. The new shape of the hair is maintained by these new disulfide links. As new hair grows out, the permanent wave process must be repeated in order to maintain the desired wave in the hair.

What Do You Think?

High-protein diets are popular among dieters. A high-protein diet that is low in carbohydrates is a fast way to lose weight. However, there are problem areas with this type of diet. Search the Internet to find the advantages and disadvantages of a high-protein diet and comment on what you think about dieting this way.

Medical Microbiology

CHAPTER **28**

Introduction to Microbiology

ADDITIONAL QUESTIONS

Multiple-Choice

Circle the best answer for each of the following questions.

1. Microorganisms that are beneficial in/on the body are called:

    a. pathogens

    b. normal flora

    c. virulent

    d. resistant

2. Departments in a medical microbiology lab can include all the following EXCEPT:

    a. parasitology

    b. mycology

    c. virology

    d. urology

3. Bacteria reproduce by a process known as:

    a. binary fission

    b. sexual reproduction

    c. phagocytosis

    d. endocytosis

4. Movement of bacteria can be accomplished by use of:

    a. capsules

    b. flagella

    c. cilia

    d. mitochondria

5. Bacterial spheres arranged in a chain-like manner are:

    a. monococci

    b. streptococci

    c. staphylococci

    d. bacilli

6. A beneficial bacteria normally found in your intestine is:

    a. *Staphylococcus aureus*

    b. *Staphylococcus epidermis*

    c. *E. Coli*

    d. *Bifidus regularis*

7. The stain test used to identify TB is:

    a. acid-fast stain

    b. Gram stain

    c. tuberculosis stain

    d. carbon stain

8. If a person presents with a productive cough and fever that have lasted for more than a week, which test would you suggest?

    a. EKG

    b. C&S

    c. CSF

    d. stool sample

9. This test determines the killing activity associated with an antibiotic:

    a. MIC

    b. KEY

    c. MBC

    d. CBS

10. This form of bacteria does not require oxygen to survive:

    a. aerobic

    b. anerobic

    c. bacteriostatic

    d. bactericidal

11. A method to identify the type of virus includes:

    a. direct detection

    b. C&S

    c. seriodiagnosis

    d. both a and c

Matching

Match the following terms with their definitions.

1. _____ *herpes simplex type I*

2. _____ RSV

3. _____ EBV

4. _____ *Varicella zoster*

5. _____ *herpes simplex II*

6. _____ human papilloma virus

7. _____ rhinovirus

8. _____ HIV

9. _____ *influenza* A, B, C

a.   chicken pox and shingles

b.   infectious mononucleosis

c.   AIDS

d.   genital warts

e.   fever blisters

f.   genital herpes

g.   croup/bronchitis

h.   viral flu

i.   common cold

Match the following terms with their definitions.

1. _____ *Giardia lamblia*

2. _____ *Entamoeba histolytica*

3. _____ hookworm

4. _____ pinworm

5. _____ plasmodium

a.   bite of infected mosquito

b.   soiled bedding or clothing

c.   can penetrate bare feet

d.   eating or drinking contaminated fecal material

e.   can cause dysentery

Short Answer and Fill-in-the-Blank

1. Staphylococcus organism stain gram _____.

2. _____ is the ability for an organism to produce an infection.

3. Hospital-acquired infections are known as _____ infections.

4. Cells making identical copies of themselves without the help of other cells is _____ reproduction.

5. The three shapes of bacteria are _____, _____, and _____.

6. _____ refers to a bunch or grape-like structure.

7. The type of antibiotic used against a wide range of organisms would be classified as _____.

8. Bacteria that is no longer affected by antibiotics is said to be _____.

9. Mycology is the study of _____.

Labeling

Label the following figure representing the various shapes and arrangements of bacterial cells.

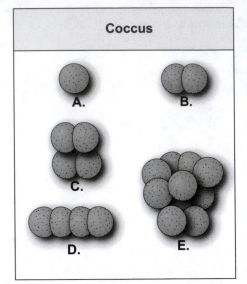

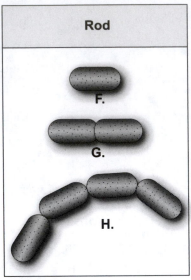

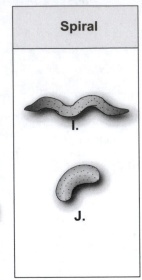

A. _____   E. _____   I. _____

B. _____   F. _____   J. _____

C. _____   G. _____

D. _____   H. _____

ADDITIONAL ACTIVITIES/LABS

1. If possible, swab various areas of your school and attempt to grow cultures on agar plates. Relate your findings to the class.

2. Plan and arrange a field trip to a hospital microbiology lab.

Extended Concepts

You have learned that the purpose of a spore is to protect a microorganism from a harsh environment. However, just how long can a spore survive? Spores found in dried plant museum samples were found to be viable even after 100 years of storage. A Roman fort that was drained and excavated contained viable spores that were approximately 2,000 years old. So if you were a science fiction writer, how far-fetched would the concept be of alien spores from other planets being found on earth or of unearthing and reviving a bacterial strain that we can no longer protect ourselves against?

What Do You Think?

What do you think about having the entire family of a person infected with active tuberculosis undergo mandatory drug therapy for up to a year? How do you weigh invasion of privacy against disease prevention and public safety?

CHAPTER **29**

Infection Control

ADDITIONAL QUESTIONS

Multiple-Choice

Circle the best answer for each of the following questions.

1. All of the following are considered PPEs EXCEPT:

   a. gloves

   b. face shield

   c. hearing protectors

   d. gowns

2. The spread of tainted blood supplies is a form of which route of transmission?

   a. indirect contact

   b. common vehicle

   c. biological vector

   d. mechanical vector

3. A tissue reaction to injury that may or may not be a result of infection is:

   a. inflammation

   b. contamination

   c. denaturing

   d. sepsis

4. The complete destruction or inactivation of all forms of microorganisms is:

   a. disinfection

   b. cleaning

   c. sterilization

   d. decontamination

5. A strong oxidizer used at a 3% solution to clean incision sites is:

   a. vinegar

   b. hydrogen peroxide

   c. quaternary ammonium

   d. alcohol

6. Ultraviolet rays disinfect by damaging the bacteria's:

   a. flagella

   b. cell wall

   c. DNA

   d. mitochondria

7. Hospital-acquired infections are called:

   a. nosocomial

   b. idiopathic

   c. chronic

   d. subacute

8. The spread of malaria by a mosquito is through which route of transmission?

   a. mechanical vector

   b. biological vector

   c. common vehicle

   d. airborne

9. Special procedures to protect yourself and your patients from contamination are called:

   a. PPEs

   b. isolation techniques

   c. standard precautions

   d. nosocomial procedures

10. Organisms that actively grow are:

    a. spores

    b. vegetative organisms

    c. denaturing organisms

    d. viable organisms

Matching

Match the following microorganisms to their disease/symptoms.

1. ____ *Staphylococcus aureus*   a.   diarrhea

2. ____ *papilloma virus*   b.   tetanus

3. ____ *Bordetella pertussis*   c.   vaginitis

4. ____ *Clostridum difficile*   d.   impetigo

5. ____ *Treponema pallidum*   e.   warts

6. ____ *Candida albicans*   f.   whooping cough

7. ____ *Clostridium tetani*   g.   syphilis

Match the following terms with their representative examples.

1. ____ direct contact   a.   a nationwide outbreak of *E. coli* in hamburger

2. ____ indirect contact   b.   infected mosquito's bite

3. ____ common vehicle   c.   kissing someone with an open sore on their lip

4. ____ airborne   d.   the use of an unclean proctoscope

5. ____ biological vector   e.   an uncovered sneeze

6. ____ mechanical vector   f.   flies walking on your potato salad

Short Answer and Fill-in-the-Blank

1. The _____ of _____ is a pathway of infection that includes transportation of a pathogen with entry into the body.

2. _____ is a general term that includes policies and procedures that monitor and control the transmission of communicable diseases.

3. _____ is a dormant and protective state of an organism.

4. _____ is the presence of microorganisms with tissue reaction.

5. Killing agent of a substance increases as the temperature _____ .

6. Immersion in boiling water for at least _____ minutes (at sea level) will kill most bacteria.

7. Acetic acid is commonly known as _____ .

8. The two most common forms of alcohol used to disinfect are _____ and _____ .

9. In both its gaseous and liquid forms, _____ is used in public pools to control pathogens.

Labeling

Label the major portals of entry to the human body in the following figure.

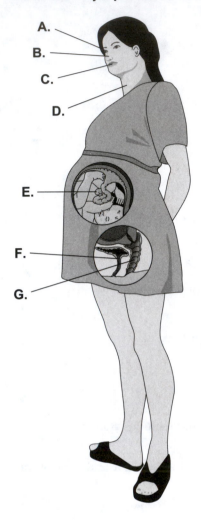

A.

B.

C.

D.

E.

F.

G.

A. _____

B. _____

C. _____

D. _____

E. _____

F. _____

G. _____

ADDITIONAL ACTIVITIES/LABS

1. Have individuals sneeze into agar plates and see what grows.

2. Review/develop infection control policies for your schools. How suitable are these for outbreaks such as H1N1?

Extended Concepts

The growing field of *epidemiology* focuses on populations and patterns of diseases. Much of the information collected by epidemiologists comes from public records such as death certificates and disease reports to public health authorities, medical records, questionnaires, and surveys. The goal of epidemiology is to define and prevent the spread of disease and assist in rapid response policy development.

What Do You Think?

What is your opinion of forced quarantine of groups of individuals who have or may possess a highly contagiously and potentially fatal infection? What are the potential legal and logistical problems you might encounter?